SEEING PATIENTS

SEEING
PATICENTS

A SURGEON'S STORY OF
RACE AND MEDICAL BIAS

With a New Preface

AUGUSTUS A. WHITE III, MD

with

DAVID CHANOFF

HARVARD UNIVERSITY PRESS
Cambridge, Massachusetts | London, England

First Harvard University Press paperback edition, 2019
First printing

Library of Congress Cataloging-in-Publication Data

White, Augustus A.
  Seeing patients : unconscious bias in health care / Augustus A. White III, with David Chanoff.
      p. ; cm.
  Includes bibliographical references and index.
  ISBN 978-0-674-04905-5 (cloth : alk. paper)
  ISBN 978-0-674-24137-4 (pbk.)
  1. White, Augustus A. 2. African American surgeons—United States—Biography. 3. Discrimination in medical care. 4. African Americans—History. 5. Medical education. I. Chanoff, David. II. Title.
  [DNLM: 1. White, Augustus A. 2. Healthcare Disparities—United States. 3. Prejudice—United States. 4. African Americans—United States—Personal Narratives. 5. Cultural Competency—United States. 6. Orthopedics—United States—Personal Narratives. W 84 AA1 W582s 2011]
  RD27.35.W53A3   2011
  362.1089′96073—dc22   2010014762

With much love
To my wife, Anita,
Who enabled me to work hard

and

To my three daughters,
Alissa, Atina, and Annica,
Who inspired me to try hard

and

To my grandchildren,
Who I trust will learn from this book

CONTENTS

When *Seeing Patients* was first published in 2011, a shock wave was reverberating through the world of health care, shaking fundamental beliefs about the relationship between doctors and patients. A few years earlier, the Institute of Medicine had published a report, *Unequal Treatment: Confronting Racial and Ethnic Disparities in Health Care*, which brought together research that had surfaced in hundreds of studies but had been so scattered it hadn't galvanized attention or created a call for action. *Unequal Treatment* documented in incontrovertible detail the fact that African Americans and Hispanic Americans received health care that was far inferior to the care provided to their white fellow Americans. Blacks received far fewer standard cardiac procedures—catheterizations, angioplasties, bypass surgeries—than whites. They received fewer kidney transplants and lung cancer surgeries, and even less pain medication for bone fractures. The mortality rate from the leading causes of death was one and a half times greater for blacks than for whites. Many of the same inequities held true for Hispanic Americans. Something lethal was going on, and it needed to be fixed.

At the time, this was a revelation to most doctors. Now, sixteen years after *Unequal Treatment*, the fact that the American health system is riven by discrimination is universally acknowledged. We now know that biased care doesn't just impact the health and lives of African Americans and Latinos. Numerous studies have shown the disparities suffered by women, gays, the elderly, and others. Thirteen groups have been documented in all: Native Americans, Asian Americans, the Appalachian poor, immigrants and refugees, those with disabilities, obese people, prisoners, and LGBT people, in addition to women, Latinos, African Americans, and the elderly. As we pointed out in the original edition of *Seeing Patients*, each specialty right down the line—orthopedics, gynecology, cardiology, oncology, psychiatry—has its own grim history of discrimination.

Today our understanding of disparate care goes far beyond the rudimentary grasp we had even a few years ago. Medical schools and professional organizations are making efforts to address the problem. There is progress. Our health-care institutions now teach culturally competent care, mindfulness, and "professionalism"—that is, a commitment to self-awareness, patient autonomy, and social justice. But we have not yet faced the true implications of inequitable care.

Inequitable care means, in plain language, that we value some lives less than others. Physicians have the ability to ease suffering, cure disease, and save lives. Unequal care means that certain groups have less access to these benefits. In other words, the human beings who constitute these groups are lower down on the scales that measure the value of life. Most physicians consider themselves to be, and strive to be, humane, compassionate, and egalitarian caregivers. Yet the statistics reveal deeply distressing discrepancies in the outcomes of those they care for—and this is true even when insurance coverage and socioeconomic factors are accounted for.

Seeing Patients tells a personal story, but it also explores some of the root causes that steer all of us, physicians and non-physicians, into discriminatory behaviors, operating beneath the surface of conscious thought and moving us without our realizing it. When I was growing up in Memphis, it was widely believed that there were significant discrepancies in aptitude and intelligence between blacks and whites. Most black doctors saw only black patients. White doctors tended to treat black patients with the condescension and patronization common in that society. The assumptions undergirding the old system have had a stubbornly persistent, if mostly unspoken, afterlife. They persist in the national psyche. They are alive in the subcurrents of our emotional lives.

In *Seeing Patients*, I look at the deep psychological processes at work and at the neurophysiology that underlies the impact of hidden emotion on rational thought.

"Feelings," neuroscientist Antonio Damasio tells us, "come first in development and retain a primacy that pervades our mental life." They "constitute a frame of reference" and "have a say on how the rest of the brain and cognition go about their business." The book shows how subconscious stereotyping, a primary function of human thinking, leads us to into likes and dislikes that stubbornly resist our efforts to erase them from our thinking. "We all make stereotypic assumptions and unwittingly make discriminatory judgments," writes David Schneider, professor of psychology and cognitive science at Rice University. "It happens with race, it happens with disability. It happens with gender, age, and physical appearance. It happens because that's the way it is: Our mental apparatus was designed to facilitate quick decisions based on category membership."

Understanding causes, no matter how intractable they might seem, is a prerequisite to addressing and counteracting them. When it comes to racism, sexism, ageism, and the other isms that constitute the litany of prejudice (and contribute so powerfully to health-care disparities), physicians are often unwitting perpetrators, but they are also ideally placed to embrace the ideals of equality and equitable treatment. This is because physicians' work is humanitarian at its very core. Doctors' whole business is to heal other human beings who, for the most part, are not close family or friends, who are to one degree or another strangers. And that—caring for strangers—is as good a definition of humanitarianism as there is. In that sense doctoring is *the* paradigmatic humanitarian profession.

Physicians are equipped by training and experience to oppose the subterranean winds that bend the mind toward the derogation of those who are different from ourselves. They see the equality of humankind in their daily practice. The suffering illness brings is the same for us all. Discomfort does not discriminate. Nor does pain. Pain is the same for you and me, black and white, Hispanic and Asian, male and female. For surgeons like myself, the equality of humankind is a living exhibit every time we operate. Once you open up the skin and look inside, everybody is the same. Underneath the surface

xii   *Preface to the Paperback Edition*

we are all brothers and sisters. The reality of the body tells you this. The reality of the spirit tells it, too. For everyone, anxiety and fear are the fellow travelers of pain and suffering; so are courage and fortitude.

Because physicians are trained to see the realities of body and spirit, they bear a special obligation to society. Their profession calls them to be models of humanitarian ideals, to be committed carriers of those values in a world so often bereft of common humanity. But doctors, needless to say, have not always taken cognizance of the humanistic and egalitarian underpinnings of their profession. The medical profession has lifted itself up only slowly from the darkness of prejudice and exclusion, as has the rest of society.

In my own life I witnessed the medical school doors just beginning to crack open enough for a tiny cohort of black students to squeeze through, of whom I was lucky enough to be one. That was not equality, but it was a gesture toward equality. The pioneering black physical anthropologist, physician, and civil rights leader Montague Cobb used to begin all his speeches, "Good morning (or afternoon or evening) my fellow humans." In his day, medical and scientific audiences rarely heard addresses from black scientists. Cobb's "my fellow humans" was a greeting, but it was also an announcement. He was acknowledging the listeners in front of him as his fellow humans; by the same token, he was reminding them that he was *their* fellow human. It was slightly startling. They weren't used to hearing a declaration like that.

The original title for *Seeing Patients* was *My Fellow Humans*. The book was (and is) an exploration of underlying causes. It seeks to reveal the mechanisms of bias and it offers solutions. It argues that physicians need to dedicate themselves to compassionate care and become fully engaged with the humanity of the patient. In this age of technological advances and reliance on sophisticated testing, that may be a tall order. But that is, as it always has been, the essence of the healing art. When we take the time to see each patient in his or her individuality, we improve outcomes and counter our vulnerability to the unseen biases we all harbor.

Seeing Patients also calls for a greater emphasis in medical schools on the humanistic side of medicine, to focus the emerging doctor on the medical encounter as first and foremost an interaction with a human being in need, rather than simply with a disease or syndrome. Both physicians in training and veteran clinicians need to know that the human dimension of practice brings enormous benefits not just to patients but to doctors. The human connection gives an additional layer of meaning to the work of doctoring. Empathy reduces stress and strengthens resilience. It enhances the well-being of the caregiver. In a profession where burnout is a pervasive problem, empathy is a powerful antidote.

When I went to medical school back in the late 1950s, there were strict quotas for black students. This was before the civil rights movement, a time when most medical schools in the country simply did not believe that a person of color might have the intelligence and diligence to become a doctor.

My story encompasses that cruel and challenging era. As a student, clinician, teacher, chief of service, and head of Harvard's Competent Care Committee, I've witnessed extraordinary changes in both the medical world's outlook and its values. But it's an ongoing process, not nearly completed yet. For so many years America inflicted immense harm on itself by providing inferior health care to those whose lives were considered of lesser worth. I've watched the medical establishment transform its thinking in that regard, but in practice we still have a very long way to go. "Of all the forms of inequity," Martin Luther King declared, "injustice in healthcare is the most shocking and inhumane." It still is, and we have less excuse for it now, because we are fully awake to its presence.

Physicians have in our hands many of the tools we need to eliminate the deep-rooted inequities in our nation's health care. We need to bring those tools to bear in our everyday practice of medicine. We need, too, to make as strong a case as possible for the importance of diversity among students and faculty at medical schools, so essential in countering stereotypes and preparing doctors for careers among a population that is itself increasingly diverse.

Seeing Patients was written in a spirit of optimism. Here is a way, it proposes, to understand the crippling and unconscionable reality of health-care disparities—and here are measures we can take to help right the ship. I thought of it as a book for doctors, but I really saw doctors as a microcosm of American society, beset by prejudices but equipped to face them and make strides toward overcoming them. The Declaration of Independence proclaimed our national commitment to the equality of mankind. The Gettysburg Address re-dedicated us to that proposition. How does inequitable health care square with our society's most basic principles? The simple answer is: It doesn't. It's possible to look at America's history as a progressive struggle to incorporate our founding ideals into the way we actually live our lives. This story, then, is a doctor's story and a health-care story, but at the same time it is an American story, of social injustice and a way forward.

The eight years between the original publication and the release of this paperback have made a difference, and not a happy one when we look at recent times. In the last few years we have seen a recrudescence of prejudice and the vilification of outgroups, a tacit and not so tacit furthering of the dark instinct for spurning and excluding those we see as different. Will this retreat from decency have an impact on bias in health care? We don't know yet, but we do know that these are bad times already for those on the wrong end of inequitable care.

It is doubly pleasing, then, that *Seeing Patients* is seeing a new light at this critical juncture. Progress toward equitable health care, like progress toward social justice more generally, requires dedication and rededication. Neither moves forward of its own accord. My sincere hope is that this new edition will contribute to both.

PREFACE

In the black South when I was a child, the first thing an adult person would ask you was: "Well, boy, what are you going to be when you grow up?" Or in my case, since my father had been a physician, "Your father was a fine man, a great doctor. You going to be a doctor like him?" My physician father died when I was eight, but some of his influence must have rubbed off, because in our playground games of cowboys and Indians I seemed to naturally want to take care of those who might have been hurt or wounded in the action.

I loved those western games, and I loved western movies, which I went to every Saturday once I was old enough. Tom Mix and Hopalong Cassidy and Roy Rogers were my heroes. Kind, peaceful men who rode into town never looking for trouble, but who inevitably found that there was evil afoot. They never looked for a fight, but when one came to them they kicked butt. That's exactly what I wanted to be like when I grew up, kind and helpful, but ready to stand up to evil and, if the occasion called for it, to kick butt.

Memphis, Tennessee, when I was coming up, was ruled by one of the segregated South's most powerful autocrats, "Boss" E. H. Crump. Under Boss Crump, Memphis was hard-core Jim Crow, a place where the races did not mix. I knew nothing about white society until, at the age of thirteen, I found myself transported north to a boarding school that accepted blacks. It was there, at the Mt. Hermon School for Boys, that I found out it was possible to actually become friends with white people.

After Mt. Hermon I attended Brown University, where I pursued my intention to become a doctor in earnest. I graduated from Brown in 1957, attended Stanford Medical School, and finished my training as an orthopedic surgeon in 1966. For many years, as a student, as a combat surgeon in Vietnam, and then as an orthopedist and teacher, I was often the only African American among my colleagues. That was sometimes an uncomfortable role, and occasionally it was more than uncomfortable. But it allowed me to experience a critical era in the evolution of American race relations from an unusual standpoint. I have had what I consider the great good fortune to be a witness to this period, from the Jim Crow South of Boss Crump to the presidency of Barack Obama.

In this book I hope to share with you something of what I have seen as a physician and as an African American. I want to try to explain how my own experiences led me to think about the biases we all have, and about medical disparities that arise from those biases and impact health care, not just for African Americans, but for Hispanics, for women, for the elderly, for gay people, and for others who differ from the mainstream. What I found surprised me. I think it may surprise you too, whether you are a doctor or a lay person. I want to describe what these disparities are, how they work to the detriment of us all, and not least, how we can go about fixing some critical parts of a mostly silent problem that so profoundly undermines the well-being of our nation.

SEEING PATIENTS

INTRODUCTION:
MY FELLOW HUMANS

There is an apocryphal story about the Ten Commandments. It's said that when Moses came down from the mountain he carried with him not ten but eleven moral prescriptions that would enable people to live together in harmony. But on his way down he accidentally dropped the tablet, and the last of God's commandments broke off and tumbled into a chasm. Moses did not feel badly, though. The eleventh commandment was the only one he was unhappy about. It had read: "Thou shalt practice no isms, neither racism nor sexism nor any other ism," and Moses believed that commandment would be far too hard for the people to follow. Looking down, God was not so sure. Moses may be right, God thought, but He had been looking forward to finding out.

—Memphis Slim

I WAS ON THE PODIUM looking out at three hundred or so of my fellow orthopedists attending the 2001 meeting of the American Association of Orthopedic Surgeons in Palm Beach, Florida. Most of the leaders in the field were sitting in front of me in the big function room at the Breakers Hotel: department chairmen, program directors, renowned clinicians, and senior research scientists, as well as their international counterparts from Canada, Great Britain, Japan, India, and elsewhere.

Good afternoon, my fellow humans. This afternoon I'll be asking you to achieve two formidable goals. The first is to change your thinking about race and the medical profession. The second is to change what you do when you get back to your

office the first thing Monday morning. In order to achieve these goals I'm going to
engage in some frank, even crusty, communication. But I don't mean to accuse,
blame, or insinuate guilt. What I have to say is in the spirit of friendship and col-
legiality. I ask you to take it that way. Call it tough love, if you will.

I wasn't exactly nervous saying this. I was a long-standing
member of the Association, and many in the room were friends or at
least acquaintances. But I wasn't exactly relaxed either. This as-
sembly was not expecting to hear what I was about to say. This
lecture, the Alfred R. Shands Jr. Lecture, was a big honor, a prestigious platform speakers almost always used to present some significant advance in bone treatment or research. Alfred Shands
himself had been a visionary leader in orthopedics, a great advocate of the importance of basic sciences in orthopedic education. I
was launching into something very far off the beaten orthopedic
track.

American biomedical science can be thought of as a beautiful and powerful fabric.
Unfortunately, this fabric also has blemishes. Today I want to trace the threads of
those blemishes. Together, we'll see how long the threads are and how thoroughly
they are woven into the fabric.

I had thought long and hard about whether to do this and, if
so, how to do it. The Shands Lecture was the featured talk at the
conference. It was a chance to get the ears of the profession's leadership on a problem that was at the top of my personal agenda, especially now that I was sixty-three years old and beginning to phase
out of my operating room career as a spine surgeon. I had been concerned about unequal treatment—disparities in health care—for
years. As an African American physician, this and other racial issues
in medicine had always been on my mind, even in the midst of a demanding professional life. But now I felt ready to really get up on the
barricades. Disparities in treatment amounted to an unconscionable and pervasive failure in the nation's health-care system. The problem demanded attention.

The unequal treatment of minorities was then—and is today—a tale of massive, unnecessary suffering among Americans who differ from the norm. Orthopedics, cardiology, oncology, gynecology, psychiatry—right down the line, almost every specialty has its own grim history of disparate care. Unequal treatment is, in its way, the last frontier of racial prejudice, all the more fascinating because so much of it is a result of biases that function below the level of consciousness, that affect even doctors who have no intention of being anything other than compassionate, egalitarian caregivers. Focusing on disparate treatment means looking at the ways stereotypes are so deeply embedded in the cognitive processes of doctors that they go largely unnoticed. It means looking at mental habits so much part of the environment that they ride beneath the surface of conscious thought and operate essentially on automatic pilot.

I thought a lot about how to present this lecture. I was going to talk to these assembled orthopedists about race and racial inequality in medical treatment—by implication, in *their* medical treatment. And some of what I had to say was pretty rough. I was obviously not going to tell these men and women—mostly men—that they were biased themselves. But I did need to tell them that their profession, of which they were the leaders, did have built-in prejudices. I needed to tell them: Look, here it is. It is not your fault. It is not my fault. But here it is. And it is our responsibility to do something about it.

I had to do this in a way that would get their attention. These were extremely busy people. They had services to run, students to teach, operations to perform, research to do, papers to read. The last thing they needed was to be told to start thinking about some issue that they had never heard of and that might have sounded peripheral to their jobs. So I had to shock them into a recognition of how deep this problem ran. But I didn't want anybody getting up and walking out of the room, either. I knew I was treading a very fine line.

Peer review journals confirm a substantial disparity in health care for minorities in America today. The infant mortality rate for blacks is more than twice that for whites. African Americans receive fewer cardiac catheterizations, fewer angio-plasties, fewer bypass surgeries, fewer kidney transplants, fewer lung cancer sur-geries. African Americans and Hispanic Americans with long bone fractures are significantly less likely to receive pain medication than whites. African Americans receive more hysterectomies, more amputations, and more bilateral orchiecto-mies [castrations]. The death rate for nine of the top ten causes of death in Amer-ica is at least 1.5 times greater for blacks than for whites.

All of this information was available in journals, from papers delivered at conferences, and from the National Center for Health Statistics. But it's unlikely that anyone in my audience had bothered to put it all together. I was emboldened to do this, not only because it was the truth and I thought the profession needed to hear it, but because my own journey as a black doctor had led me to it. I felt I had a responsibility to do it, an obligation. When I was putting the lecture together I thought: Who else is going to tell them this? And if someone else does, will they listen? I thought it would be significant that they hear it from a minority person who was one of their own. Hearing it from a white peer would be important, but hearing it from me would have more of a shock value. I didn't have any illusions about where this might go, just that it was better than nothing. And, for this audience, the baseline on this subject was nothing.[1]

Professor Jack Geiger at CUNY Medical School has reviewed 600 citations docu-menting disparities in the treatment of African Americans and Hispanic Ameri-cans. They suggest strongly that physician bias and stereotyping, however uncon-scious, is the cause. Are you shocked by this? Are you shocked by this image?

I clicked the remote and projected a slide onto the screen: a photograph of a black woman in a long dress hanging by her neck from a rope. I had taken it with permission from a book entitled *Without Sanctuary: Lynching Photography in America.*

This woman's name was Laura Nelson. She was thirty-five. In 1911 she was hanged from a bridge outside Okemah, Oklahoma, alongside her fourteen-year-

old son. How can we understand something like this? Does it have any connection to Dr. Geiger's observations? Can history help us answer this question?

This was not an easy slide to look at. *Without Sanctuary,* the book I found it in, reproduced photographs of American lynchings originally gathered by James Allen for a traveling exhibit cosponsored by Emory University. I grew up myself in the segregated South, at a time when lynchings like this were still taking place. I hadn't been able to steel myself to actually go to the exhibit. But I had bought the book.

Over three-plus decades of writing and teaching I had given hundreds of lectures on the biomechanics of the spine; I had a whole professional lifetime of talking about bones and joints to audiences of orthopedic surgeons and neurosurgeons. Like every other veteran speaker, I had learned, consciously and unconsciously, to register my listeners' reactions from their body language: their interest, their resonance, their skepticism, their approval. Looking out at this audience, I was not seeing a lot of resonance. What I was seeing was a lot of discomfort. What I was seeing was some element of, Why is he talking to us about this? I was sensing a little resentment out there, and maybe even some anger.

So, can history help us understand the connection between the lynching of Laura Nelson and her son in 1911 and the often unconscious but sometimes conscious prejudice that results in unequal health care? Why don't we begin with Plato and Aristotle, the fathers of Western science. Plato and Aristotle laid the foundation for so much of Western thought. They also, unfortunately, laid the foundation for racial bias.

Plato can be said to have originated the Great Chain of Being theory, which dominated Western thinking about the structure of the world and the relationship of its elements for almost two millennia. Aristotle's ideas of the gradation and continuity of the different types and classes of living organisms filled out the concept. The

Great Chain of Being is, as its name indicates, a hierarchical scheme. Lower leads to higher. In living organisms lower species lead by steps to those that exhibit some degree of reason. In this realm, as one eighteenth-century writer put it, "Animal life ... in the dog, the monkey, and the chimpanzee ... unites so closely with the lowest degree ... in man that they cannot be easily distinguished from each other. From this lowest degree in the brutal Hottentot, reason advances through the various stages of human understanding."[2] The seventeenth and eighteenth centuries were replete with searches for the missing link between ape and man, a link that was frequently found in the supposedly apelike African.

Now allow me to share with you a quote from Galen, the Greek physician whose thought was the leading influence on medical theory and practice up through the Renaissance. There are, Galen wrote, "ten specific attributes of the black man. Frizzy hair, thin eyebrows, broad nostrils, thick lips, pointed teeth, smelly skin, black eyes, furrowed hands, a long penis, and great merriment ... That merriment dominates the black man ... because of his defective brain, whence also the weakness of his intelligence." Galen lived in the second century A.D. Now let's skip 1,600 years to Carolus Linnaeus, the eighteenth-century Swedish botanist and physician whose Systema Naturae first framed the principles for defining the genera and species of organisms. He too designated Africans as lascivious, inferior, and apelike.

I only had forty minutes here, not anywhere close to the time it would take to even mention the racial theories of more modern, almost equally consequential scientists: Louis Agassiz, for example, perhaps the greatest and most influential of nineteenth-century American naturalists, who argued that blacks are a separately created and inferior species; or Ernst Haeckel, the eminent German biologist and physician who coined the phrase "ontogeny recapitulates phylogeny" and led the fight for the acceptance of Darwin's theory of evolution. Haeckel too believed blacks are inferior. They are, he thought, a step on the evolutionary ladder between orangutans and northern European whites.[3] Agassiz, magisterial as his work in zoology was, still

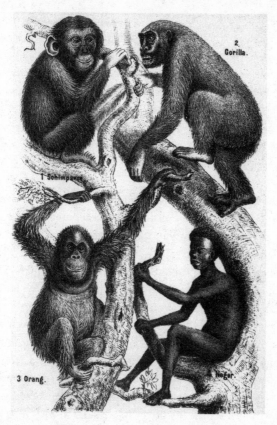

The 1872 edition of Ernst Haeckel's *Anthropogenie* contains this racist illustration of evolution. Reprinted with permission. Image #336734 © American Museum of Natural History, New York, NY.

subscribed to the notion of creationism and rejected Darwin's theory. Haeckel embraced Darwin and believed that creationism was pure superstition. Blacks caught hell from both of them.

Because a picture is worth a thousand words, I clicked the remote and showed the orthopedists a second slide, taken from Haeckel's *Anthropogenie*.

Amid this historical hopscotch there is the central phenomenon of pseudoscience. Pseudoscience embodies a variety of measurements or examination of body parts and dimensions by learned scientists as well as by the unlearned. Wherever differences between black people and white people were found, they were taken to confirm attributions of inferiority to people of color. Phrenology and craniometry are examples of pseudosciences. Phrenology involved reading bumps on the skull to determine character. Craniometry measured skull size to determine intelligence. These endeavors, needless to say, also demonstrated the inferiority of both black moral character and black intelligence.

Finally, to drive home the point of how "science" and racist cultural beliefs have reinforced each other, I noted the case of Saartjie Baartman, the European name bestowed on a South African Khoi house servant who was transported to England in 1810 by a ship's surgeon for study and display purposes. Baartman exhibited pronounced steatopygia—the accumulation of fat in the buttocks—and also elongated labia minora, unusual by European standards and known initially as "Hottentot Apron." She was subjected to the minute attention of a team of researchers led by the French Academy of Science biologist Etienne Geoffroy Saint-Hilaire, who declared her to be a lower form of life, inferior, sensual, and related to the ape.[4]

I didn't have the time, or perhaps the heart, to describe for my fellow orthopedists the history of Baartman's display as "The Hottentot Venus" first as a pseudoscientific exhibit, then as a sideshow-style entertainment, or how spectators paid to crowd around her near-naked form, staring close up at her so-called deformities, or how after her early death her body was dissected by George Cuvier, the founder of comparative anatomy, and her brain and vagina displayed at the Paris Museum of Man until 1974. "These races with depressed and compressed skulls," Cuvier wrote, "are condemned to a never-ending inferiority. [Saartjie's] moves had something... reminding [one] of monkeys ... and a way of pouting her lips in the same manner as we have observed in orang-utangs."[5] But I did have time to project a slide showing the naked Baartman being ogled by Europeans.

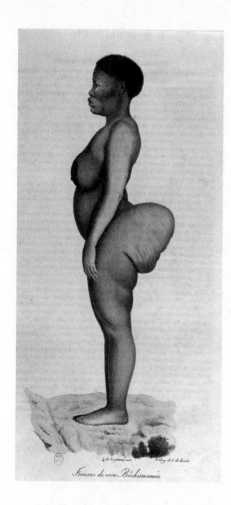

Saartjie Baartman (also known as "The Hottentot Venus, Bushman woman") from "L'Histoire Naturelle des Mammiferes" by Etienne Geoffroy Saint-Hilaire (1772–1844) and Frederic Cuvier (1773–1838), 1824 (color litho). The Bibliotheque Nationale, Paris, France/Archives Charmet/The Bridgeman Art Library.

It hardly needed saying that Saartjie Baartman was not treated as a human being. She constituted the most dramatic and emotional pseudoscientific exploitation of race I knew of. Displayed first as a sensational semihuman, semianimal curiosity, then as an exhibit in a leading anthropological and ethnographic museum, her case drove home how science and pseudoscience conspired, not just over centuries, but over millennia, to ingrain in the Western mind the assumption of black inferiority. Doctors and other scientists were responsible in part for its formulation and promulgation. They theorized about it, and they acted on it.

Dr. J. Marion Sims (1813–1883) was the father of gynecological surgery. Dr. Sims performed multiple surgical procedures on female slaves to develop his rectovaginal fistula repair operation and other surgical techniques. "In one case," he wrote, "I purchased my patient in order to operate." He operated on the slave Anarcha at least thirty times. Dr. Sims used no anesthesia, just opiates. He believed blacks did not have morals or perceive pain like whites.

A striking classical antecedent of Dr. Sims's use of slaves for experimentation was the vivisection experiments of third-century B.C. Greek physicians Herophilus and Erasistratos of Alexandria, who "laid open men whilst alive—criminals received out of prison from the kings—and whilst these were still breathing observed parts which beforehand nature had concealed."[6] These were prisoners, the lowest rung of society, forerunners of the blacks and convicts whom American medical scientists used so frequently for their own experiments.

Here's more of our medical heritage. In the nineteenth century's lexicon of Negro diseases we find the term "dreptomania," defined as "diseases causing Negroes to run away." Another disease, "furor sexualis," was defined as "black man's attacks, like bulls and elephants in their intensity . . . the price . . . syphilis." In terms of Negroes' physiological peculiarities we find that "Blacks have larger penises and breasts than whites—signs of indolent and unbridled sexuality . . . Blacks engage in social relationships with apes. Apes captured and enslaved blacks and abused them sexually."

But it is hardly necessary to go back to former eras to find parallels to Dr. Sims and his notorious experiments. The American medical research community regularly resorted to using blacks as either involuntary or unaware research subjects in painful and potentially lethal studies of vaccines and other therapies. The most infamous of these was the Public Health Service's Tuskegee Study, which sought to determine the natural course of syphilis through an observational study in which almost 500 black men suffering from the disease were left untreated without their consent from 1932 to 1972.

The Tuskegee and other medical experiments, as dramatic as they were, only touch on the vast scope of unequal treatment that has characterized the relationship between African Americans and the medical community from slavery times onward. Inferior medical care (or no care at all) has accompanied inferior treatment of black Americans across the board from the earliest colonial period through slavery and segregation—all of it impelled by the propagandistic identification of blacks as something less than fully human.

But while this poisonous fiction of black inferiority has informed the Western mind-set, at the same time we, as children of the American Revolution, are imbued with democratic, egalitarian ideals. They were the founding principles of the country, and without a doubt, we as a people subscribe to them. How, then, do these two powerful currents interact?

The answer is: Not easily. By the end of the eighteenth century, industrial slavery had been a fact of life and an economic pillar of America's growth for almost two hundred years. The high ideals of Revolutionary democracy, captured so memorably in Jefferson's Declaration "We hold these truths to be self-evident, that all men are created equal," had a hard time competing with the economic demand for slave labor. Jefferson, himself a slave owner, had, it's fairly clear, a guilty conscience about the divide between the ideal of equality he espoused and the financial needs his planter way of life dictated. "I tremble for my country," he wrote, "when I reflect that God is just: that his justice cannot sleep forever."[7] Patrick Henry too was a slave owner, the same Patrick Henry who famously pronounced "Give me liberty or give me death" in the Virginia House of Burgesses. "Would anyone believe," he wrote to a friend, "that I am Master of Slaves of my own purchase! I will not, I cannot justify it."[8]

It was a lot easier for slave owners to see slaves as not qualifying in the all-men-are-created-equal category if they in fact were a little less than human, a little more like apes. And this was the prevailing mind-set. Or possibly because blacks were cursed by God, the common interpretation of the story of Noah's son Ham by slavery apologists who appealed to the Bible for justification.

These toxic myths are now, thank goodness, in our past. But the background noise of black inferiority has not by any means disappeared. It is part of our cultural ambience, and doctors are as subject to it as everyone else. Disparate care is the legacy of several thousand years of conditioning. Escaping from conditioning this deep is no easy matter. But if we are to confront it at all, awareness is the absolute prerequisite.

Why do we want to correct this unconscionable reality suffered by some of our fellow humans? Because we are a nation and a people with high humanitarian ideals, the ideals of the Declaration of Independence, of the Pledge of Allegiance ("with liberty and justice for all"), and of the Gettysburg Address (a nation "conceived in liberty and dedicated to the proposition that all men are created equal").

High humanitarian ideals first, but also enlightened self-interest. Safety, for one thing: In the less healthy portion of the population, there is almost always a residue of communicable diseases that can and do affect the majority of the nation. Cost, for another: A large proportion of disparate care is crisis care, which is more expensive. It costs far more, for example, to perform an amputation than to treat a diabetic's infected ingrown toenail. National success in the global marketplace, for a third: Nations that will do best in the future will be those with a healthy workforce. In 2000 the World Health Organization ranked America's health twenty-fourth in the world, just above Cyprus and not far ahead of Cuba. Our minority population that suffers from disparate care is 28 percent of the total. By 2050 minorities are projected to be 47 percent of the population. If we do not correct health disparities, where do you think the United States will stand in the rankings by then?

At this point I trust that you are excited, motivated, and enthusiastically asking, What can I do? Allow me to share some general thoughts. We, as physicians, can be societal leaders in facing racism. We have been educated to address cancer, amputations, paralysis, and death with strength, sensitivity, equanimity, empathy, and rational good judgment. We are capable of extending these skills to the manage-

ment of racism and other isms. We physicians do not generally face clinical problems with guilt, anger, denial, or rationalization. We face them analytically and constructively. We can face racial problems in medicine the same way.

NOBODY DID WALK OUT. A friend of mine said later that no one dared; everyone else would have thought that person a racist. That may or may not be too harsh. Afterward there was a decent volume of applause, and then the room emptied out, as it ordinarily would. I didn't sense that I had made a roomful of converts. But a number of people stayed to talk. Tony Rankin, an African American leader in the orthopedic community, came up and shook my hand. "Thanks," he said. "That took guts." A few of the visiting international doctors came by to smile and shake hands. From them I got a sense of camaraderie and mutual understanding. Being outsiders, they were aware of our history of racial issues but didn't feel conflicted or tense about them.

When the little knot of people had mostly thinned out, Joseph Buckwalter, the Association's president, stopped to talk. "Gus," he said, "you have to publish this in the *Journal of Bone and Joint Surgery*." Joseph Buckwalter was a longtime friend, but this was not something I expected to hear. Shands lectures were not ordinarily published; in fact, when I looked it up I found that none of them had been published. I don't think anyone had ever criticized the profession in this way from such a podium, so it hadn't even occurred to me to publish it, especially not in the premier professional journal. The *JBJS* went out to 35,000 orthopedists.

But, encouraged by Buckwalter's suggestion, I submitted the paper to the usual peer review process, and it was accepted for publication. For that to have happened there had to be some willpower behind the decision, and a significant level of responsiveness. Once you publish something like this, no one can hide from it. People can and do refer to it. They don't have to spend an hour and a half trying to retell an argument, they just cite a reference. They send it to their friends. They discuss it. If they've been thinking along these lines already, an article can galvanize them into some kind of action. If they haven't been thinking about it, they start to.

It had taken a long time for my colleagues to get to a point where they were at least prepared to listen. Of course, it had also taken a long time personally for me to get to where I was; a long time and a long evolution in my own experience of race generally, starting out in segregationist-era Memphis, Tennessee, and extending through my tenure in the world of medicine, which had been my professional home now for so many years.

1

IT TAKES A VILLAGE: MEMPHIS

If anyone's niggers is going to fly, mine is.

—E. H. "Boss" Crump, political boss of Memphis, Tennessee,
upon hearing about the Tuskegee program
for black combat pilots in 1941

EDWARD HULL CRUMP ran Memphis for half a century, which included the time I was growing up. But in some ways "Boss" Crump was not the typical Southern boss politician. He thought colored folk were all right, provided they did what he told them to do. They could vote, for instance—as long as they voted for him. His chief black political operative was Lieutenant George Washington Lee, a successful businessman who had fought in World War I as one of the army's first black officers. Growing up, I thought "lieutenant" was the highest rank the army had.

Memphis was segregated then, strictly Jim Crow. The city had a thriving black middle class, with families like the Walkers and Fords and Gibsons, but the white world did not mix with the black and the black did not mix with the white. Except maybe at the nightclubs and brothels on Beale Street, where blacks were often the entertainment and whites were the entertained.

One of the many places blacks and whites did not mix was in the world of medicine, a world I was born into, literally. My father, Augustus White, Jr., was a doctor who had graduated in 1929 from Meharry Medical College, founded a decade after the Civil War by the Methodist Church because "the difficulty of securing proper medical attention for the colored people was very great and the

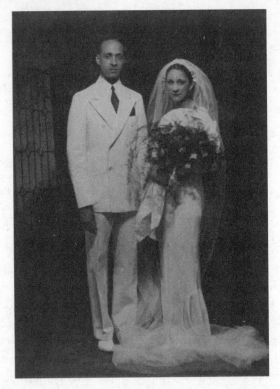

Wedding photo of Augustus A. White, Jr., and Vivian Odetta Dandridge, 1934. From the AA White Family Collection.

mortality among them alarming."[1] Dad came to Memphis as house physician at Terrell Memorial Hospital, where I was born in 1936, and where we lived, in an apartment above the main entrance, until I was four.

"Old Bo," he used to say, taking me to stand between his long legs as he sat in his chair. "Old Bo, your dad is so proud of you. I want you to be a good boy and a strong boy, and I want you to always remember to take care of your mother." That was something I did remember, most especially after he died suddenly, probably of a heart attack—we never knew for sure—when I was eight.

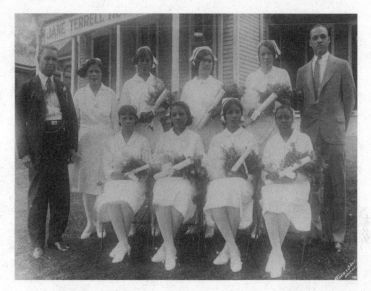

Dr. N. M. Watson (left) and Dr. Augustus A. White, Jr. (far right) with a class of graduating nurses in front of the Jane Terrell Memorial Hospital, Memphis, Tennessee. Photo courtesy Hooks Brothers Photography.

After that I did take care of my mom, as best I knew how, just as she took care of me. Together, she would tell me, the two of us were her "big team."

My father's death when I was so young meant that most of my relationship with him ended up being my relationship with his reputation. In the black South, at least while I was growing up, when an adult met a little kid, right after "hello," you, the little kid, would hear, "Well, boy, what are you going to be when you grow up?" Or, in my case, "You going to be a doctor like your dad? Your dad was a fine man. He was a fine man, a great doctor. You should be proud of your dad." This continued for years after he passed on. So I was regularly reminded of whom I was supposed to emulate, which I think did inspire me and inculcate in me the idea that being a doctor was something a person could be extremely proud of.

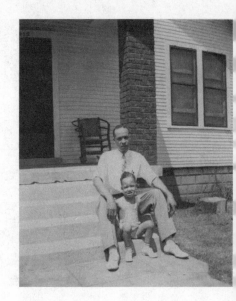

At age three with my father on the steps of the family home, Memphis, Tennesee. Photo by Vivian White.

His death also meant that Mom and I very quickly found ourselves downsized. From the hospital, we—Mom, Dad, and I—had moved into a little white two-bedroom house on Polk Street. But when he died it turned out that the house, our car, and whatever clothes we had in the closets constituted the whole of our net worth. (Years later I actually found the probate report: my mother's share of the estate came to $527.96.) As a result, Mom went almost instantaneously from middle-class homemaker to working-class single mother. She was a graduate of LeMoyne College, where she had majored in English, and also of the Henderson Business College, where she had learned secretarial skills. And since it was easier to find work as a secretary than as an English major, that's what she did, becoming a secretary at LeMoyne before eventually getting a teaching position at the city's Frederick Douglass High School.

That was on the work front. On the living front, we had to sell the house and move in with my mom's sister Addie and her husband, C. S. "Doc" Jones—"Doc" because he was a pharmacist who owned his own drugstore business. Aunt Addie and Uncle Doc were family-oriented, warm-hearted people, so living with them quickly came to seem perfectly natural. My maternal grandmother, Lucy Dandridge, lived there too. In fact, I moved into her bedroom, onto a fold-up cot. My mother, as I remember, slept on the sofa bed in the living room. "C'mon, big team," Mom would say when it was time to get up for school. "C'mon, big team. Let's go get 'em."

I cannot recall my father ever talking to me about race, but Doc, who became more or less my surrogate father until my mother remarried, was, I think, more attuned to those issues. Doc eventually built his own drugstore, but when I was young the pharmacy was on Thomas Street, in a building owned by a Jewish family, the Wieners. Mr. Wiener's dry goods store took up one half of the building and Doc's drugstore the other half. In Memphis, black and white kids were just as segregated as their elders. They didn't go to school or church together, they didn't play with each other, they hardly interacted at all—which was my experience too, except that I knew Mr. Wiener's kids, Marty, who was my age, and Barbara, who was a year or two older.

Since I spent time hanging out with Doc at his store and the Wiener kids spent time at their dad's, I used to play with them on occasion, mostly with Marty, less often with Barbara. But one day I was out back with Barbara—Marty was not there for some reason. We were playing in the yard there with whatever toys we could rustle up, and somewhere in the course of our game we decided we needed a horse, or a mule. And being an agreeable child, I volunteered. I got down on all fours and Barbara mounted up and began to ride, shouting the occasional "Giddyup, mule! Giddyup!"

But while I was bouncing along down there, very satisfied with my mule impersonation, Doc came to the back screen door, probably attracted by the giddyups. "Hey, partner," I heard. "Come in here for a minute." When I got inside he was beside himself, so choked up he could hardly speak. I had never seen him like that. I was worried that something might be happening to him. "Boy," he said, "don't you ever be any kind of mule for white folk!" "Oh," I said. "We were just playing." But that didn't satisfy him. "It doesn't matter,

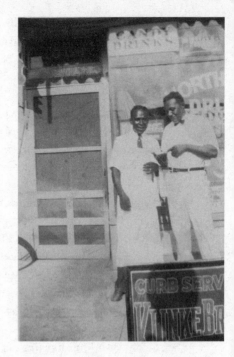

Dr. C. S. Jones (Uncle Doc) on the right with deliveryman in front of Doc's Northside Drug Store, Memphis, Tennesee, circa 1933.
From the AA White Family Collection.

boy. You've got to have more pride than that. Don't you never, ever be no mule to no white people!" He said that like he meant it.

By then I was beginning to register more about race from other sources too, one of which was the *Pittsburgh Courier*. The *Courier* served as the national black newspaper; it was sold all over the country, including in Memphis, where at the age of eight I was a *Courier* newsboy. The distributor would drop off a stack of papers on the corner where Doc's pharmacy was, and I'd take them around the neighborhood. I delivered papers to subscribers first, then I hawked the leftovers, yelling, "Extra, Extra! Read all about it!" which I knew was what you were supposed to shout, since I had seen it in the movies. "Extra! Extra! Big NAACP Convention in St. Louis! Read all about it!"

Now, the *Pittsburgh Courier* was a great paper. It was printed on dark pink newsprint, which attracted attention all by itself. It had cartoons and a regular column by Langston Hughes writing under the pen name Jesse B. Simple. It advocated for "the rights of colored people," and during the war came out with its "Double V Campaign," V for Victory (America's) Abroad and V for Victory (ours) at Home. Photographs accompanied stories, just as you would see in any newspaper, pictures of dignitaries shaking hands and car accidents and newly dedicated buildings. But once in a while there would be another kind of photograph, a photograph of a lynched black person, a person hanged, or shot. Painful, scary pictures that made me angry. When something like that was on the front page, I didn't want to take the newspaper around. I didn't even want to handle it.

The family used to wonder why we didn't have our own lynching victim over an incident that had happened to an aunt of Grandma Lucy's back in slave days. Grandma Lucy would tell the story of her Aunt Hattie, a tall, dark woman she remembered well. According to Grandma Lucy, Hattie had been picked on and mistreated by a vicious overseer one time too many, which had caused her to lose her temper and her mind both and pick up her hoe and drive its blade into that overseer's neck, almost but not quite killing him. We were not a violence-prone family, but we were all proud of Aunty Hattie. We wondered why they hadn't killed her for that, though; the main opinion being that the plantation owner must have known her as a hard-working, decent woman and the overseer as a brutal thug, and so had let Hattie off with a warning that she had better steer clear of attacking anyone else.

I believe that something of Hattie's need to resist got passed down to my own mother, Vivian, and her sister Addie. The custom in the South in those days was that white people called black people by their first names, John or Charles or William or sometimes just "boy." It didn't matter how old you were; you could be sixty and your white interlocutor far younger, and you would still be a boy. Or a "gal," because the same went for women. Meanwhile, the black person in this exchange would call the white person Mister or Miss or doctor or sir or whatever term of respect was appropriate.

But Vivian and Addie refused to accept this and they developed their own method of guerrilla warfare. If one of them was shopping at a store and had taken all her purchases up to the checkout counter, that's when the resistance demonstration was likely to commence. Maybe the checkout clerk would know who she was, or see her name on a check, or might need to ask for a name and address. And if that checkout clerk had the temerity to say "Addie" or "Vivian" ("Addie, is this your current address?"), that checkout person would hear, "Oh, I am *so* sorry you called me 'Addie.' My name is *Mrs.* Jones. And I do need these items here, but now I can't have them, because I do not shop in a store where I am not respected." And she would walk out.

Vivian White and Addie Jones did not feel inferior to anybody, and they were not about to be treated as if they were, not if they could help it. I picked up on that feeling early; it would have been hard not to in that family. Of course, other than Marty and Barbara Wiener I had no firsthand experience of white people, so I didn't actually know how they might treat you. I did hear about it quite a bit, though, not that it was all completely negative.

The black middle class in Memphis consisted mostly of businessmen, doctors, lawyers, and teachers, but head waiters and bell captains were at least on the margins; their incomes were often substantial. These waiters and bellmen were service people, but they were professional service people. They knew their jobs and did them well, and that included understanding human nature, especially the male pride part. They knew, for example, how to greet their customers. "Mr. Jones, so nice to see you back, sir." And the diner or hotel guest would feel recognized, acknowledged. So yes, the waiter or bellman served white folks, but at some level he was the one in control, he was the one manipulating the situation. It was part of his professionalism; he gave good service and he was paid well for it.

Now, I did not want to be a waiter or a bellman when I grew up, but I knew that people with those jobs were respected. They had an obvious dignity about them. So serving others never seemed to me to have anything degrading about it. Doc taught that lesson too, when I

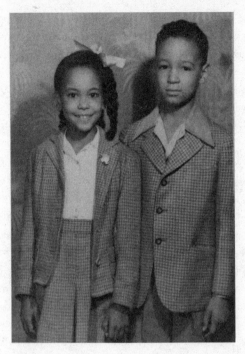

With my first cousin, Alphanette Price, both age nine, 1945. From the AA
White Family Collection.

started working in his drugstore. You were polite. You treated people
with respect, no matter who they were; treat them well and they will
treat you well. And when I was in sixth grade I got a job as a kind of
waiter myself. A carhop waiter at a Memphis drive-in movie theater.

One of my friends worked at the drive-in, and he asked me if I
would like to work there too. They needed help, and you could make
some money there, not in wages—there were none—but in tips. The
drive-in was on the other side of Memphis. Getting there meant a bus,
a trolley to the end of the line, and a mile-and-a-half walk. But it was
interesting. Drive-in movies were popular, but blacks were not allowed
into them in Memphis, so there was a big curiosity factor. Besides that,
the job appealed to my acquisitive instinct. So I took him up on it.

The work consisted of picking up Cokes and popcorn from the concession man and selling them to the customers in their cars. This I did with a significant level of enthusiasm, maximizing my interactions, and my tips, in every way I could think of. My customers not only got their Cokes and popcorn, they got a friendly face, an upbeat greeting, and a free windshield wash with the bottle of Windex and the cloth I kept in my back pocket. The tips added up fast. And, while schools in those days did not teach sex education, the drive-in provided demonstration lessons in every variety of romantic interaction that might be carried on inside a car, so that was an additional benefit of sorts.

I did get to see a lot of white people in that job. I also, not infrequently, got asked a peculiar question by these white people. They would look at me and say something like, "By the way, what nationality are you?" Marty and Barbara, the only white people in my previous experience, had never asked me that, and it took me a bit to understand that I was really being asked what race I was. My light skin color—both my parents had light complexions—made them curious. And then there was my manner, which I like to think was forthright and not subservient. I might be "colored," but maybe I was just some kind of foreigner, Cuban or something. Or could I actually be white?—it was a little hard to see in the dim drive-in lighting. In which case there could be serious offense taken if they asked whether I was black or not. Better to be on the safe side. So, "What nationality are you?" "American," I'd answer, a little confused. I mean, what else would I be? Then, after I picked up on it, I'd say "Negro," which I was proud of, just like Mom and Aunt Addie and Uncle Doc were. So that was my nationality for the summer. Negro.

It wasn't all politeness. The concession man who dispensed the Cokes and popcorn to us wasn't too happy with how much money we were making, most likely more than he was. I also figured change fast; working Uncle Doc's cash register had given me a facility for it. And since we carhops bought the refreshments from the concession man, then got reimbursed for what we didn't sell, we were constantly figuring balances, which he was slow at and I wasn't. As the concession man's resentment grew, he began calling us "darkies," as in, "You darkies better get a move on," or "Which of you darkies is going to be working tonight? That darkie who was here yesterday or some other darkie?" And that usage spread to the concession man's white co-workers.

I have got to tell you, this was a very upsetting thing. It made me and my friend and the two others working with us angry. So we made up our minds to do something about it, though we knew we'd have to tread carefully. We decided to call them "Nabisco boys." After all, if we were darkies, what did that make them? Crackers, right? That is, "Nabisco boys," which gave us satisfaction without stirring a hornet's nest, we thought, since they didn't understand what we were talking about. They'd say, "You darkies," and we'd say, "What is it, Nabisco boy?"

But maybe we weren't quite as clever as we thought, because although they might not have known what "Nabisco boy" meant, it was pretty clearly not some kind of respectful superlative. And one night as the tension was ratcheting higher, a car pulled up opposite us as we were walking the mile and a half to the trolley stop after work. Three or four white boys or men were in the car, screaming undecipherable curses at us. Then one of them stuck a rifle out the window and started shooting, except with the first report it was obviously not a rifle but a BB gun. We ran like hell, including one upper-crust black society kid whom we had just brought out to work that day. A black society kid who was so scared he began to stutter. "L-L-L-L-Lordy mercy," he stammered as we took off down the road, the BBs zipping around us. "L-L-L-L-Lordy mercy, Lordy mercy, Lordy mercy." If I weren't so panicked myself I would have had a laughing fit. Like us, he was twelve years old. He had never met a white person before. This was his introduction.

Fortunately, they didn't chase us, so we got out of there safely, except for two of the guys who had gotten painfully zinged. Back home, though, Mom and Aunt Addie practically had a fit. My friend was not going out there again; the society kid probably didn't want to lay eyes on another white person the rest of his life. But Vivian

White and Addie Jones were not going to take this kind of thing, and after some discussion they made it clear that I was not going to take it either. The next day they drove me out to work and had a talk with the ticket lady, who managed the drive-in, and the concession supervisor, who I was sure was one of the men in the car. This cannot happen, they told them. They didn't know who was responsible, but it must be stopped! I had done nothing wrong and I had to be able to work there safely and no one should be allowed to bother me. That should be crystal clear to everybody! And people should understand that if such a thing did take place again, they would be back!

I didn't know at the time that this incident would stay with me the rest of my life, but what a lesson it was. They were formidable. And, interestingly, the drive-in manager responded positively. She wasn't happy about what had happened, and she assured these two powerful black women that this kind of thing would not be repeated and that I would be safe. And nothing further did happen. I recruited a couple of other friends and we worked there the rest of that season and the next season too.

Vivian and Addie provided me with a world of strength. I knew I was not just loved, I was looked after. But they were not the only ones who threw their protective shield around me and made me know that I was a person of worth, a person of potential. Addie, like Vivian, was a high school teacher, as well as being a guidance counselor and later in her life a writer. She, Doc, and my mom were college graduates; my dad too, of course. They were part of Memphis's college-educated, black professional and business class, which constituted its own close-knit society, with institutions—fraternities, sororities, clubs, camps, and networks—that connected them with the educated black elite of other cities around the country.

Mom and Addie were Delta Sigma Theta. Doc was Phi Beta Sigma. Dad had been an Alpha Phi Alpha. The common denominator of these groups and others like them was education. Their aim was to nurture achievement and pride. In a way, they constituted a national village, with values its members were expected to maintain and goals they were expected to reach. A child growing up in this class did not grow up alone. He or she grew up understanding that people were watching, that people had expectations. In the Memphis part of this national village that I was raised in, you learned, by osmosis as much as anything, that you had obligations and responsibilities. You were cared for and encouraged; your accomplishments were celebrated—that was the adults' side of the bargain. Your side of it was to get educated and make something of yourself. That was how the race advanced, and you were a part of that effort.

Growing up black in Memphis, that was me, but hardly just me. And hardly just middle class. The same message was conveyed to all Memphis's African American young people by the city's segregated schools: Douglass and Manassas and Booker T. Washington. It was as if the teachers in those schools had all gotten together in some kind of mass training and decided on a message. And that message was education, education, education. Education was how you were going to rise up from where you were to where you should be. Education was how you were going to show the white world who you were and what you were capable of doing, what *we* were capable of doing. Education was going to drive forward our right to equality that we had been struggling so hard for so long to achieve.

The teachers especially looked out for those they thought had potential. And if it seemed to them that some capable student wasn't working hard enough, they would come down hard. "You've got to do your work! You hear me? You better do this!" They'd jump on you. They'd ride roughshod over you. They'd whack you on your hands with a leather strap. "You want to spend your life pushing some white baby around? That what you want to do with your life?"—this to some intelligent girl. "Boy, you planning to be some field hand? You think that's what God gave you a brain for?"

Education was part of the program. The other part was pride. We learned about Booker T. Washington; Toussaint Louverture; Benjamin Banneker, who surveyed Washington, D.C.; Frederick Douglass; W. E. B. Du Bois. We'd have assemblies where they would preach Negro history and pride. Mary McLeod Bethune spoke at one of them—I remember her well. One of the greatest African American educators, she had started a school for girls in Florida that eventually evolved into Bethune-Cookman University. She fought for civil rights, she registered people to vote, she became a close friend of Eleanor Roosevelt and an adviser to Franklin Roosevelt on racial issues. Mary McLeod Bethune was a force of nature. She was a large, powerful woman with a broad face. She started her speech, "I'm black and ugly . . . but I *know* something."

IN MEMPHIS, BLACK PEOPLE were constantly pushing against the white world that beset them in so many ways. But we had our own color issues too. Light and dark made a difference. It's a classic problem in the black community—not that I was aware of it on that level as a kid. I was aware of it on my level, though.

When I was playing in the neighborhood, my light skin color sometimes made me a target. Other kids would mess with me. Sometimes I'd be "Red," or "Yellah," or "White Folks." I'd try to fire back something, but a lot of times it would be older or bigger kids, and I'd just have to swallow it. I wasn't ostracized or anything; some kids were black, some were brown, some were light, and we all hung out and played together. But the teasing was hurtful, especially when I was younger, in second or third or fourth grade. "You don't have anything to feel bad about, honey," my mother told me. "You didn't determine what your color is. God determined that."

About a year after my father died, my mother started going out with, and then married, Charlie Tarpley, a biology teacher and coach at Booker T. Washington High School. That made a big difference in my life, not least because one of the sports Charlie Tarpley coached was boxing and because I soon became probably his youngest boxing student.

Charlie Tarpley's good looks and buoyant personality made him a popular man. He had been in the army and had a million stories to tell about his experiences there and on the road and in sports, all of which sounded fascinating and adventurous, at least to me. Charlie exuded energy. He'd bounce around while telling his stories, enacting what had happened as well as describing it. He liked to play tricks with baseballs or basketballs, spinning them on a finger or making them disappear behind his back. He'd play around, showing me his judo and boxing moves. And because he was a gifted coach with a sure feel for kids, he pretty quickly recognized that I could benefit from some instruction.

Soon enough he was teaching me how to throw a punch, how to move and duck. He'd demonstrate the almighty jab, the right cross, the left hook, the uppercut, the bolo punch, putting up his palms for me to use as targets and telling me all the while about Joe Louis's killer right or Sugar Ray Robinson's feared bolo.

After some months of this I found that my fighting skills were becoming gratifyingly more proficient than those of my playground adversaries, which gave me a pretty good handle on the teasing business about my light skin. Not that I won all my fights, and there weren't all that many of them to begin with. But at least I could stand up and make a point.

My boxing career ended up by going beyond the playground too. Apparently Charlie saw something in my reflexes, or maybe just my eagerness, that put him in a more serious frame of mind. One day as we were gliding through our usual fun combinations he said, "Okay, now you need to start preparing for the Tri-State Boxing Tournament." This was the major regional Golden Gloves–level tournament for ages eight or nine through high school. I can't say I was ready for this, or aspired to it, or ever even thought about it. But I did end up competing, first in the "ant-weight," eighty-pound limit division, then the following year as a "mosquito-weight."

I didn't win, and there was no doubt that my future wasn't going to be in the ring. But I learned a lot, and I did compete some later on in camp and in college. Thanks mainly to Charlie Tarpley, I learned how to take a punch and give one, which meant a lot to me. Boxing was standing up for yourself, which was why Joe Louis was so adored in the black world. Here was a man who could stand up, who could beat the best the white world had to offer. Boxing, of course, didn't carry that kind of meaning for me. But I did respond to the idea of standing up for myself. It gave me confidence to know I could do that.

It wasn't just boxing, though. I loved sports altogether—the sandlot football and baseball we played, and just the rough and tumble of being a kid in a neighborhood full of kids. Every Saturday a bunch of us would also go to the movies to see whatever cowboy film was playing, Tom Mix, or Hopalong Cassidy, or Wild Bill Hickok. We'd mainly go to the all-black movie houses, the Savoy and the Ace, rather than to the segregated theaters where you'd have to sit up in the balcony. I loved those cowboy heroes. I loved how they knew how to stand up for themselves. They'd come into town on their white horses, peaceful and certainly not looking for trouble. Some of them would even sing. But they'd invariably find that there was evil abroad and that people were being oppressed. They'd try to avoid a fight as long as they could. But when it became necessary to finally stand up, they kicked ass.

I knew, beyond a shred of doubt, that that was what I wanted to be like. That was my ideal. I wanted to be kind and helpful, like they were. I wanted to be peaceful. But if it came down to it, I wanted to face up to evil and kick ass too.

ONE OF MY FRIENDS in Memphis was Walter Gibson, who, if not a genius, was certainly close. Walter's father was a distinguished biology professor at LeMoyne College who had been a good friend and fraternity brother of my father. Walter's mom was a teacher. As black educators, the Gibsons knew that there were several elite white prep schools in the country that accepted black students, one of which was the Mt. Hermon School for Boys up in Massachusetts. And having a gifted son, namely Walter, Dr. and Mrs. Gibson made arrangements to send him there.

I was in the kitchen one evening with Mom and Aunt Addie while they were making dinner, and at some point Aunt Addie said, "By the way, do you know that Walter Gibson is going to be going to Mt. Hermon next year? That's a prep school in New England." This possibly (but possibly not) off-hand remark was followed by some talk about what a good education they provided up there. Then there was a long pause, after which my mother said, "Tell me, how would you like to go to prep school?"

After another long pause, not knowing anything about anything, I said, "Yes, I'd like to go." After all, Walter was going to prep school, so why not me?

That was quite an inspiration on their part. And an aspiration. I'm sure the Gibsons' situation put it in their minds. They were positive a prep school education would be superior to what I would get in Memphis's public high schools. But they didn't know much more than that—the fact was that if any black kid from Memphis had ever gone to a high-class white prep school before, none of us had ever heard about it. As they started to look into these schools, or at least into the ones that were known to accept blacks, they found that the tuitions were astronomical. Mom's teacher's salary was a little over a thousand dollars a year, and some of these schools cost almost as much or more than she was making. By chance, the only one that might possibly be affordable turned out to be Mt. Hermon School for Boys. The reason their rates were so much lower was that each Mt. Hermon student had to do ten hours of work a week, cleaning, maintenance, kitchen—some kind of real work. Mt. Hermon believed this was part of the educational experience. It also lowered their costs by a considerable margin.

Given Mom's meager resources, it was still a struggle, even with Addie and Doc pitching in what they could. But they all finally figured they could just about handle it, so I filled out the application, took the required Wechsler Bellevue IQ test, and waited to hear.

The Mt. Hermon response came back in a thick envelope, which any student today would understand instantly as an acceptance. Without any experience of such things, we were on pins and needles as we opened it up, to find that I had, in fact, gotten in. There were all sorts of instructions and advice too: what kind of warm outer clothing I should bring (Massachusetts was cold), the sports jackets and ties I would need (to conform to the dinner dress code), the vaccinations that would be required. And one other medical item. In order to attend the Mt. Hermon School for Boys, one had to be circumcised. Was I circumcised? the form asked. If not, my family should arrange for the procedure prior to registration.

We did not know if this was something required of all applicants by all prep schools or if this was special, a rite of passage specific to the circumstances of admission for students like myself. In any event, it seemed that if I was going to be allowed to go to school with white people and receive a superior education, I would have to undergo a ritual that, as far as we knew, was a biblical injunction concerning male babies of the Jewish religion.

That part of the Mt. Hermon admissions package precipitated quite a bit of discussion and thought in the family, and I know for a fact that no one thought about it more than I did. We also enlisted the services of Dr. Quintus Cooper to help with our considerations. He was a young doctor and family friend who had rented the second floor, above Doc's drugstore. I had even helped him move some of his furniture and equipment in.

In the end it was decided that despite the strangeness of this requirement, a prep school education was certainly worth it and that we would conform. That is, I would conform. And Dr. Cooper would implement the conforming.

The operation took place in his office with just the two of us present. With my subsequent experience of medicine and surgery, I feel safe in saying that this circumcision was one of the first, or more likely the very first, such procedure Dr. Quintus Cooper had ever performed. I watched as he first administered a local analgesic with a hypodermic syringe. After that he was, again on the basis of my later surgical experience, quite tentative in his exposition of the procedure, which, as I recall, lasted two hours instead of the ten minutes or so such things normally take. Yes, it hurt. And yes, I remember him having some difficulty placing the stitches and adjusting their length. He took, I would say, extreme care. Extreme and lengthy care. But overall, I would rate it a good job. Even though his initial injections of analgesic went a little too deep and punctured the wall of the urethra, which healed up after a few days and left no lasting damage. But for those few days, whenever I urinated I watched, fascinated, as the urine stream exited various places in addition to the proper one, so that the performance resembled nothing so much as somebody watering flowers out of a shower-type watering can.

I never mentioned that to anyone, though. I was just happy to know that I had completed all of Mt. Hermon's entrance requirements. Together with Walter Gibson, I was now ready to plunge into the world of white education.

2

SCRUB NURSE

I can with truth and sincerity declare that I have found amongst the negroes as great a variety of talents as amongst a like number of whites; and I am so bold to assert, that the notion entertained by some that the blacks are inferior in their capacities, is a vulgar prejudice founded on the pride of ignorance.

—Anthony Benezet, eighteenth-century Philadelphia Quaker,
teacher, and founder of a school for black children

AT THE AGE OF THIRTEEN the term "culture shock" was not in my vocabulary. Had it been, I might have been culture shocked-out, considering the chasm between what I knew—the black side of segregated Memphis, Tennessee—and what I had now gotten myself into: the white Mt. Hermon School for Boys on the bank of the Connecticut River in the classic New England countryside of northwestern Massachusetts. Walter Gibson and I roomed together. Other than us, there were three other "colored" boys in our class of 120 or so. Among the students at Mt. Hermon, black faces were few and far between. Among the faculty, there were none at all.

Being cast into this sea of white people was a little disorienting. One problem was that Mt. Hermon's idea of time didn't exactly jibe with my idea of time. Mt. Hermon was tightly structured. There were schedules, and you had to stick to them. But for some inexplicable reason, I found that knowing where I needed to be and getting there on time was a real challenge. I didn't know why that was; at home I didn't seem to have problems like that. But up here I started accumulating "tardies." Was it just that I didn't know my way around yet, or did white people really keep time differently than we did? It made me wonder.

The music was different too. Back home there was always music, and all of it with that big beat. Gut bucket blues, R&B, and rock and roll. When you turned the radio on or put a coin in a jukebox, there was Howlin' Wolf or Muddy Waters or B. B. King, the "Beale Street Blues Boy." Or early rockers like Little Richard, Fats Domino, and Bo Diddley. Memphis was the place. We had the Beale Street jazz clubs and Sam Phillips recording black music—"race music," as it was called in those days. We had WDIA with DJ Reverend Gatemouth Moore and WHBQ with the slightly insane Dewy Phillips playing all our music. But the boys at Mt. Hermon weren't listening to anything like that; they didn't even know it existed. Instead they liked Dixieland and bland-sounding popular tunes, the most unhip music imaginable, at least in my book.

Still, all and all I didn't feel as out of place at Mt. Hermon as I might have at Andover or Exeter or one of the other bastions of the white elite. As far as my family knew, Mt. Hermon was an upper-class white prep school, in the sense that to us all prep schools were white and upper class. But in reality, Mt. Hermon was different. It had been founded in 1881 by Dwight L. Moody, the great evangelical revivalist preacher of those days, who also founded the Moody Bible Institute. Moody's original idea was to educate young people who might make good workers for his movement—poor boys, foreign boys, boys of slave parents; he wasn't particular. Over the years, the founding evangelical spirit of the place had more or less dissipated. But the school's culture retained other Moody hallmarks. His educational motto was all over the place: "Educate the head, the heart, and the hand." Boys were expected to be hard working, humble, responsible, respectful, and (on the sports field, anyway) competitive. I was pretty much ready to go with that whole program, not least the competitive part.

My plan for getting along at Mt. Hermon was simple. I'd just keep my head down, watch what the others were doing, and try to do the same. You were supposed to carry yourself humbly and say "sir"?

I carried myself humbly and said "sir." You were supposed to do your ten-hour-a-week job without complaining? I did it, and I didn't complain either—even though my first assignment was cleaning toilets. You were supposed to study hard and give a good account of yourself in the classroom? I did my best. If this was how white people acted, that was okay with me. It didn't seem all that different from how black people acted. Maybe race wasn't such a big issue here, I thought. Especially given the issues that did almost wholly monopolize my attention. One was that I absolutely had to get myself "classified." A second was that I more than absolutely had to get myself onto the freshman football team.

Somehow Mom, Addie, and I had missed the part in the school information packet about getting "classified." Or maybe it wasn't there but was only announced once new students arrived on campus. Becoming a "classified freshman" was what happened after the first two marking periods, assuming your grades were good enough. If they were, you were accepted as a legitimate, bona fide, matriculated person. You were classified. You had passed your first hurdle.

Football was another story. Everyone at Mt. Hermon played sports, and in the fall, football was the sport to play. Back home I had been a pretty good sandlot football player. My stepfather, Charlie Tarpley, had drilled me, especially on pass catching, and that, together with a high degree of motivation, put me right in the thick of our playground games. There was nothing in the world I loved more than football, nothing. At Mt. Hermon I knew I wouldn't be able to make the cut for the top group of freshman and sophomores. At five foot two and 113 pounds, I wasn't anywhere near big enough. But I just had to make the second level, the so-called Ivy League. Ivy League players all got pads and uniforms. I needed to get that uniform. Those poor kids who didn't make Ivy League were shunted over to soccer, an unthinkable fate.

As the first marking period drew to a close, my only problem on the classification front was our Old Testament Bible class. I don't know if I had a strong point at that stage of my educational career, but if I did, it definitely was not reading. And it most definitely was not reading the Old Testament, with its antique, King James English—as attested by my grade for that period of 35. All my other grades were okay, Bs and Cs, but that 35 was going to put me under. I had to shape that up, which I truly buckled down to do, and I ended up passing the course, barely. But that barely was enough to get me classified.

On the football field, when we had finished all the tryouts I was sitting with the fifty or sixty other boys who hadn't made the select group, all of us biting our nails with anxiety, watching as the coach made his decisions about who would play in the Ivy League. Those he pointed at took off across the field as if they were spring-loaded, sprinting toward the gym, where a uniform awaited. I was one of the smallest of those sitting boys. I had also managed to catch only about half the passes thrown to me during practice. I was desperate. Doom was staring me straight in the eyes. Until, Yes! Coach's finger pointed at me, and I took off toward the gym like a bat out of hell.

It's possible coach was moved by the look of utter need and determination in my eyes. I wanted so much to be successful. For myself, of course. And for my mom, who wrote to me almost every day, her letters full of love and confidence in me and my ability, as she saw it, to be a great student and do big things. I badly needed to make her proud, to come home with some kind of accomplishment under my belt.

When Walter and I did go back home for Christmas vacation we found that it wasn't just our parents who were interested in how we were doing; we were something of a news item in Memphis. We were the boys who had gone off to that white school in Massachusetts. The *Memphis World,* our local black newspaper, did a big article on us, complete with a photograph that had us looking like we were the co-winners of a contest for innocence and naïveté. Like me, Walter had been immersed in the challenges of Mt. Hermon life. But here we were, back in our home village, where it was apparent that both our successes and our failures were being noted. Like it or not, we were *representing.*

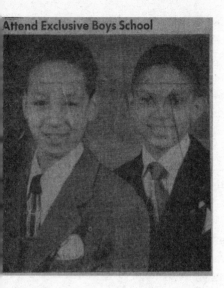

Attend Exclusive Boys School

The caption to this 1950 photograph from the *Memphis World* reads: "Two Memphis students [I at left, Walter Gibson at right, both age thirteen] are headed back to the prep school at Mt. Hermon School in Massachusetts after three weeks' spring vacation spent with their families in Memphis."

The rest of that first Mt. Hermon year I kept my head down and followed the plan, putting one foot in front of the other and giving every challenge my best shot. My grades got better, I joined the wrestling team, I got promoted from toilet cleaner to floor sweeper—all positives. All my life I had imbibed those family lessons about how I was just as good as anyone else; that is to say, I was just as good as white kids. In retrospect, Mt. Hermon was a kind of testing laboratory for that theory. I was measuring myself, competing. I had a natural appetite for competition that I'm sure was considerably intensified by all those expectations. Mt. Hermon boys were supposed to be humble, never to strive after recognition, but to accept it with modesty if by chance it happened to come their way. Humility was a key value at Mt. Hermon, and I did my best to assimilate it. But I had a strong desire for recognition too.

A lot of that came out on the athletic field. I arrived at Mt. Hermon as a scrawny thirteen-year-old; one of Mt. Hermon's star varsity football players, a brother no less, had watched me play as a freshman and pronounced me a gutsy kid but too "light-in-the-ass."

But by the time I was a senior my genes and hormones were doing their duty. I had sprouted up to six foot two, a good size to carry onto the football field, where I made varsity, and the wrestling mat, where I wrestled in the 177-pound class and was even elected captain.

By then I had also found a sport I loved, to my astonishment, even more than football: lacrosse. This wasn't a game anyone in Memphis had ever heard of at the time. But if we had heard of it I think we would have enjoyed it. American Indians had invented it as a way to toughen up young warriors. They sometimes used it as a substitute for warfare; contending villages would play against each other in games that covered many square miles, lasted for days, and typically produced many casualties. Lacrosse as played in the prep school leagues had been substantially modified from those early days, but it hadn't lost its rough side. It was the kind of game someone like Jim Brown, among the toughest football players of all time, could love. It complemented football nicely, except that people could hit each other with sticks.

I mention Jim Brown because he was not only a Hall of Fame football great, he was also a legendary lacrosse player in high school and college, and not least because I got to play against him when I was Mt. Hermon's starting center midfielder. Although I played sports through college, facing up to Jim Brown my senior year at Mt. Hermon was probably the pinnacle of my athletic career. Brown at that time played for Manhasset High School on Long Island. He was already very nearly his professional football playing size of six foot two, 230 pounds, and he was already famous for his extraordinary athletic prowess. Red Smith, the great sports writer, said that for "explosive violence" in a "package of undistilled evil," there was no one like him. Manhasset was a public school, but every spring they toured New England, teaching the prep school teams what lacrosse was really about. One of the stops on their tour of destruction was Mt. Hermon.

Since Jim Brown was Manhasset's center midfielder and I was Mt. Hermon's, we were going to be playing opposite each other. And since he was already practically a mythological figure, I realized beforehand that I could never match up against him playing both offense and defense, which is what midfielders are supposed to do. His speed and power would just overwhelm me. So I decided I had only one goal for the game: to keep Jim Brown from scoring on me. To save my strength, I wouldn't really play offense. And on defense I wouldn't try to muscle him or bang him—I'd just stay locked up with him. I would be in his face and in his way every moment. I'd be on him like white on rice, or in this case, White on Brown. Jim Brown ordinarily scored six or seven or eight goals a game, sometimes more. I didn't want him scoring one goal—not on me, anyway.

We lost the game, of course. But somehow I managed to win my own little game within the game. The man did not score on me. As I said, it was the pinnacle of my athletic career. Afterward I introduced myself while the Manhasset players were having lunch in our dining room. "Hi," I said, "I'm the guy who played against you at center mid. I just wanted to come over and say hello." Jim Brown did not possess a warm and fuzzy personality. Later in life I met him several times and he was cordial, in his fashion. But the best that could be said of our postgame encounter was that he did not encourage conversation.

That was a bit of a disappointment, but that aside, Brown, as I said, was already a phenomenon, and I had unbounded admiration for him and for black athletes in general. People like Joe Louis and Sugar Ray Robinson, Satchel Paige and Jackie Robinson, Jim Brown and Muhammed Ali were heroes to a black community that badly needed heroes. In the thirties, forties, and well into the fifties and even the sixties, most fields of endeavor were closed to African Americans. Sports and music were two areas where blacks were able to excel, and the people who did, especially when they did it in relation to whites, bore a lot of pride and hope on their backs. They were magnificent—not just because of their exceptional talents, but because they possessed the spirit and willpower to punch their way to the top against a world full of obstacles. They embodied optimism and confidence; they inspired people. I took them to heart personally. We all did.

For me, as for many black kids, sports had an emotional dimension that went well beyond the physical side. I'm not sure my Aunt Addie appreciated the full importance of that when she sent me a packet of information about a special scholarship available at Morehouse College. This was during the second half of my freshman year, when I was still only thirteen. I was just getting to feel at home at Mt. Hermon, but Addie was pushing Morehouse hard.

Morehouse was (and still is) one of the leading traditionally black colleges. And Morehouse, it seemed, had a connection with the Ford Foundation, which administered a special test. Those who did well enough would be admitted to Morehouse on full scholarship when they finished their first year of high school. It may have been that Morehouse had a special program for youngsters who came in via this test. I didn't know that. What I did know was that Addie's enthusiasm for Morehouse was boundless. Morehouse was the school for me, no question about it. Winning a scholarship there would be important financially; it would also bring with it all sorts of prestige and visibility, on top of the educational advantages. She was thrilled and excited about this opportunity. I should be too. I should plan on going there. It was spring vacation and Mom was away, but Addie was Mom's older sister and she was used to calling the tune. Besides, she was absolutely sure my mother would feel the same. Dr. Gibson, Walter's father, certainly did. Walter was definitely going to take the test.

The problem was that I didn't share Addie's enthusiasm. Morehouse might be a great place. I was sure it was. But after looking into it, I found that they didn't have a junior varsity football team. At Morehouse it was varsity or nothing. For me, that would mean . . . nothing. As young and light in the ass as I was, I could forget about football. I could forget sports altogether. And there was just no way I was going to do that.

In the end I did take the test, mostly to satisfy Aunt Addie, and I did well enough to qualify for the scholarship. But I refused to go, even after I was invited to come down and tour the college. Morehouse was beautiful, but there was no question; I was staying at Mt. Hermon.

That was a road not taken. I often wondered afterward how my life might have been different had I gone to Morehouse along with Walter, who scored brilliantly on the test. But the truth was that Mt. Hermon was giving me just what I needed at that point in my life. I was growing to love my studies, history, philosophy, and literature—but especially biology. I took an advanced course in that subject and something just clicked, which made me more certain than ever that one day I was going to be a doctor. I loved sports, and playing on Mt. Hermon's teams, I found out that I was a pretty good athlete. I loved music, and singing in the Mt. Hermon choir, I discovered Bach and Handel and Mozart. I don't know if they actually displaced Muddy Waters and Howlin' Wolf and B. B. King for me, but singing the Hallelujah Chorus or listening to Bach's Toccata and Fugue in G Minor played on the chapel's great organ put me into a kind of ecstasy. I even got a lot of satisfaction out of my various student jobs. Maybe not the toilet-cleaning job or the floor-sweeping job, but after that I became a waiter, which carried a lot of prestige with it. And after that I became a faculty waiter, which was as high up on the prestige ladder as you could get. Mt. Hermon reinforced my self-confidence in a dozen different ways. At graduation I was given an award for having won varsity letters in three sports and a plaque that told me I had "come a long way *to* Mount Hermon, and had gone a long way *at* Mount Hermon." I don't know who was prouder of that, my mom or me. In my senior year, when I began thinking hard about colleges, I felt sure that I could measure up wherever I went.

WHEN IT CAME to choosing a college I had three criteria. First, did it have football, lacrosse, and wrestling? I wanted to compete in all three. Second, did it have a good premed program? And third, how did it treat Negroes?

Using these criteria, I quickly narrowed down my search to three. My first choice was Middlebury College in Middlebury, Vermont. Middlebury played my sports, they had a good premed program, and they most likely didn't treat black students poorly—though that was conjectural since, according to my informal grapevine, they didn't have any black students.

I understood why when my classmate and fellow waiter Bob Chutter invited me to his home in Rutland, Vermont, for Thanksgiving. Bob's family lived in a beautiful old New England house, and they were as welcoming as could be. But in Rutland I froze to death day and night. I went to sleep shivering and woke up shivering. Then I shivered till it was time to go to sleep again. And Rutland was south of Middlebury, which meant Middlebury was even colder. I thought East Brookfield, Massachusetts, had inured me to winter, but apparently not. Vermont was obviously just too frigid for soul brothers. I didn't even complete the application.

Another choice was Amherst College, where they also played my sports and had good premed courses. According to the Amherst catalog, there was one scholarship available for a Negro student. On the one hand, that was encouraging. On the other, it might have meant that they took only one Negro student per year. Whichever, I decided to apply. But I didn't win the scholarship. And I wasn't accepted either. Which left Brown University. Brown had good athletics, highly regarded premed studies, and, my grapevine informed me, they not only took Negroes, they treated them well. Four or five each year. Never more, but never fewer either. In the entering class of 1953 they took five, of whom I was fortunate enough to be one.

Looking back, with all the complexity involved in the college admissions process, it was amazing that Brown during the fifties consistently admitted four or five African American men and Pembroke (Brown's all-female sister school) two or three African American women each and every year. The quota system was obviously in full operation. I don't know if there was still a Jewish quota in those days; I don't think there was. But there most certainly was a black one. Equally amazing is that we, Brown's African American students, didn't feel affronted by this plain discrimination. Quite the opposite; we felt happy to be at a place so liberal that it accepted Negroes at all.

Whatever Brown's institutional racism might have been back then, I personally came into college understanding that white people could be your friends. As a thirteen-year-old freshman at Mt. Hermon I had had no way of knowing that. But by the time I graduated from there, I knew that whites were more or less just like everyone else. In that regard, my concept of racial equality was pretty far ahead of Brown's, at least as embodied in the university's admission policies. But white students were also confronting the ingrained racism of their institutions, among them the brothers of the Delta Upsilon fraternity.

As the fraternity rush season began that first semester, DU brothers began showing up at my dormitory room to introduce themselves and talk to me about the advantages of being a Delta Upsilon. DU was a kind of academic jock house, with a strong representation of scholar-athletes. The DU brothers had a bit of a serious, gentlemanly air about them. They had fun, but if a Brown freshman was looking for heavy-duty drinking and rowdiness, DU was most definitely not for him. I was a football player, a wrestler, a lacrosse player. I was no genius, but I was serious about my studies, friendly, but not in any way a party animal. I probably fit the DU description as well as anyone. Except, that is, for the hard-to-overlook fact of my skin color. Brown University had no black fraternity, and no Brown fraternity had ever had a black member. In rushing me, the DU brothers were doing something unprecedented. In its own way, it was a courageous act. I'm sure they thought long and hard about their decision to invite me in. I found out later that they had even discussed it with some of their alumni. I certainly thought long and hard about whether to accept their invitation.

My concern was the other brothers, my black brothers. There were only sixteen of us on campus, a small, tight little community. Most of us hung out together. We'd get together in one of the guys' rooms and listen to jazz for hours, telling jokes, talking abut girls, our courses, sports—and race. We were the "club members," as we called ourselves. Retaining my credibility with this group as a loyal black guy and stalwart soul brother was a high priority. But they knew DU was rushing me. How was my joining a white fraternity going to square with my club brotherhood?

"Hey, Gus." (This was from Ted Parrish, a club member from the inner city of Springfield, Massachusetts, considerably darker than I was. He had been reading about race in his sociology class, and now we were in one of our bull sessions.) "Hey, Gus, about this skin color thing. You know, they say whites are more accepting of Negroes with light complexions. There's supposed to be an inverse relationship. The darker you are, the more difficult it is to be accepted. The lighter you are, the easier to integrate. What do you think about that?" A test, of course. I was the lightest person in the room.

"Yeah," I said. "I can believe that. That's probably true. That's probably why they're asking me to join DU."

Pause. Silence. Nothing.

I had said the right thing. If I had said, "No, whites think of us all the same way. That has nothing to do with why they're asking me to join DU," I'd probably have been dead in the water. As it was, I wasn't aggrandizing myself or defending the DU white guys. Besides, who knew? I didn't want to think so, but maybe it had been easier for them to take me because of my complexion.

I believe, even in retrospect, that my DU brothers actually took me because they thought I fit in and because they thought it was the right thing to do. This was 1953, the year *Brown v. Board of Education* was argued and the beginning of desegregation in schools and restaurants throughout the South. The army had been desegregated in 1947, the same year Jackie Robinson broke the Major League color barrier. By the time I entered college, Martin Luther King had already started his civil rights work. Rosa Parks was going to come along a year and a half later. The spirit of integration was building. At Brown, DU took the lead in breaking the fraternity color barrier. I think they were proud they were doing it, and they should have been.

Meanwhile, for the black community at that time, the idea of equality more or less meant the idea of integration. Integration wasn't just a good thing, it was what we were fighting for, to become an integrated part of American society. That was what equality meant. So breaking the fraternity color line was a big deal. DU thought it was doing something good, and I thought I was doing something good. Truth be told, I even felt a little touch of heroism, as if I were the Jackie Robinson of fraternities.

I didn't get any Jackie Robinson kudos from anyone, though, and the fraternity didn't get kudos of any kind. What we got was a lot of trouble. Two years later my DU brothers voted me the chapter's president-elect, and as president-elect I was one of the two designated representatives to the national convention, certified under the name "Gus White," no racial qualification mentioned. But it was known that the Brown DU chapter had admitted a Negro, and eventually the National discovered that the Brown chapter's delegate, Gus White, was that very same Negro.

That summer before the convention I began getting messages from National officers by phone and mail telling me in a semidiplomatic way that my presence might provoke something they wouldn't be able to handle. They were concerned for my safety. Wouldn't I consider withdrawing as Brown's delegate in favor of someone else? I told them I wouldn't. My brothers had elected me and I wasn't going to unelect myself. Besides, I wasn't worried; some of my Brown brothers would be with me. So no, I was planning to come and hoped to participate actively.

I thought that my membership, and my forthcoming presidency, was a signal manifestation of black/white goodwill, and I wanted to continue that effort at the convention. I didn't know if the National was envisioning a big race riot or something. I didn't think that was likely—the convention was going to be held in Middlebury, Vermont, not Little Rock, Arkansas. But I felt ready for whatever might happen. I thought that my presence would make a statement, and I wanted to make that statement. This situation was going to be my own contribution to racial progress. Not a major-league-baseball-size contribution maybe, but still, definitely a contribution.

My high hopes, though, went down in flames when I received the following telegram: THE MIDDLEBURY CHAPTER REGRETS THAT DUE

TO CIRCUMSTANCES BEYOND ITS CONTROL, AND WITH THE CONCURRENCE OF THE COMMITTEE ON ADMINISTRATION, IT IS NECESSARY TO POSTPONE THE DELTA UPSILON CONVENTION AT MIDDLEBURY UNTIL 1957.

That shocked me; it hit me hard. I could hardly believe it. I felt we had been defeated and slapped down. *I* had been defeated and slapped down, and *they* had won. After a while my anger tamped down a bit, but the whole thing left me with a bad feeling. To make matters worse, at the next convention that did take place, the Brown chapter was censured for "committing an unfraternal" act, namely, admitting "a person not socially acceptable to the rest of the fraternity." And sometime subsequent to that, the Brown chapter disaffiliated itself from the National fraternity.

To skip quite a few years ahead for a moment, in 1986, the National fraternity somehow came across the history of this affair and decided to do what they could to rectify it. They tracked me down, which wasn't hard to do since by that time I was a member of the Brown University Board of Trustees. The National fraternity president, Judge Terry Bullock, contacted both the Brown chapter and me personally, frankly apologizing for what had happened back then and asking for a full reconciliation.[1]

The fact was, that experience hadn't left me with any indelible scars. I had chalked it up to the times and hadn't given it any particular thought over the years. But I felt gratified to be contacted. And I learned that in the interim Delta Upsilon had become an organization that actively promoted diversity and racial harmony. Not only that, after several meetings with Judge Bullock, me, a number of my DU classmates, and John Robinson (Brown's then dean of students), the National fraternity decided to make a contribution to Brown's Investment in Diversity Fund, a scholarship endowment to enhance the university's effort to increase its own diversity. Nobody mentioned the word "reparations," but I must admit that that was the way I thought of it.

I don't believe the ironies in this situation escaped anyone's notice. In my student days Brown had kept its African American population to a severe minimum. Thirty years later, the university's dean of students was himself African American and Brown was making a major effort to recruit African American students. The Investment in Diversity Fund had been conceived by Harold Bailey, a fellow African American trustee. I had been asked to serve as its first chairman. If some Brown student from my day had fallen into a thirty-year coma and had just woken up, he would have thought he was still dreaming.

To cap it off, Judge Bullock invited me to speak at the next DU national convention, held in St. Louis. I did, and my speech was received with a long standing ovation, after which the delegates formally rescinded the 1956 resolution censuring the Brown chapter for its "unfraternal act." I can tell you that the delivery and celebration of justice does feel good to all concerned, no matter how long you might have to stick around to see it.

But all this is getting very far ahead of the story. Brown, of course, was a lot more than pictures in black and white. I did get to wrestle some and play lacrosse, although I dropped out of wrestling after my sophomore year to concentrate on my studies better, and lacrosse was only a club sport so, though I played, it didn't take much time. But football—football was another story.

FOOTBALL I PLAYED right through all four years. Though I loved lacrosse, football had a special meaning for me. Football was the first sport I knew anything about. My Uncle Arnett had told me that he and my dad played when they were in college. In Memphis, football was the major sport, the one everyone talked about and everyone played, or wanted to play. Then there was Charlie Tarpley, my stepfather, who coached me on how to catch passes and how to fake and get away from tacklers. I liked that. I took pleasure in bringing down a pass and taking off at full speed. I loved faking some would-be tackler out of his jock, leaving him standing there looking or sprawled out on the ground. I had an adolescent boy's macho enjoyment of hitting people and knocking them down, or trying to keep them from hitting me and knocking me down. I loved to make clean tackles, get my arms around somebody's two legs and bring him down with a quick half-roll. I brought all of that along with me to Brown.

"Football teaches you to make a commitment," said my end coach, Joe Restic, who later coached for many years at Harvard. He had been an end himself, like me, offensive and defensive. "When you're out at the end, you have all those people coming at you. You've got to commit. You've got to stand up and be counted." That resonated with me. I really did want to stand up and be counted, physically, intellectually, racially, every way I could. That was a part of me, a need I had that just cried out to be satisfied. And you couldn't stand up and be counted any more visibly than out there on a football field playing end.

I was ready to sacrifice for that, and football for a premed was definitely a sacrifice. Premed meant studying like a maniac and getting the best possible grades. Premed meant taking science courses with afternoon labs that often got in the way of practice. You just

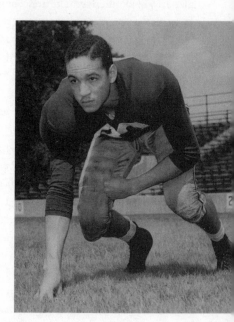

Offensive and defensive end, Brown University varsity football seasons, 1954–1956. Photo: Office of Sports Information, Brown University.

had to miss one or the other, but you still had to excel at both, and how in the world were you supposed to do that?

One way I found was by majoring not in any of the hard sciences—biology, chemistry, physics—but in psychology. Psychology had its fair share of labs, but fewer than I would have had as a hard science major. So I did have to miss football practices, but not quite so many. I also fell in love with psychology, in particular with experimental psychology, which was Brown's strong suit. So I did study like a maniac, but in my psych courses, anyway, it always seemed more like fun than work. I also had the great good fortune to cross paths with Professor Anthony Davis, who taught the course in child psychology I took as a sophomore.

This was a large class. I had done well on a couple of papers and exams but wasn't aware that I was standing out in any way. But after the lecture one day, Professor Davis stopped me on my way out. "May I speak to you for a moment?" he said. "I like your work. You're a good student. I'd like to talk to you about some of your plans. Why don't you make an appointment with my secretary to come and see me."

Well! That wasn't just unexpected, it was jolting. The fact was that, though I had had good teachers at Mt. Hermon, even some I idolized, no one had ever said such a thing to me before. And the Brown professors? I was a sophomore, and I was still mostly in awe.

Needless to say, I made an appointment as fast as I could. When I told Professor Davis that I was planning to go to medical school, he asked if I'd thought much about doing an honors thesis. No, I told him, I had not. I did not tell him that I wasn't even aware there was such a thing. But, of course, there was. An honors thesis meant doing an independent research project together with a professor, and in my case, if that's what I wanted to do, it would be with Professor Davis himself.

Now the fact is, if Professor Anthony Davis had not tapped me on the shoulder, and had not by so doing increased my level of confidence by several magnitudes, and had he not subsequently guided my work and mentored me, I would still have gotten into medical school. But I would not have experienced what it means to develop the methodology for an original piece of research; I would not have worked with a senior professor to carry out an experiment, identifying problems and devising solutions; I would not have actually published a paper (together with Professor Davis) in a leading refereed journal as an undergraduate; and I would not have had the kind of ongoing advice and encouragement that any aspiring student would die for, and that was so significant to this aspiring student in particular.

When it came time to apply to medical school, I selected seven that I thought looked especially good, my top choices being Yale, Harvard, and Stanford. These applications were enough to raise anybody's anxiety. Medical schools were famously selective, and grades were the primary criterion. Mine were good; I had been on the dean's list every semester after my first and I was graduating with high honors in psychology. But they weren't superlative. They might have been better if I had had more time to study. But as it was, there was football (I was actually invited to the Chicago Cardinal training camp), there was the fraternity, there were my four years on the student council, and there were my jobs as a waiter in the cafeteria and a proctor in the dormitory, which had all added up to a full plate. And that didn't include the time I was spending with a beautiful brown-skinned, hazel-eyed Pembroke coed who was taking more and more of my attention—not that I regretted that in the least. Not that I regretted any of it. Except for the jobs, which I needed for money, nobody had twisted my arm to do those things. And given all that, I was proud of my grades. But would they be good enough?

I liked Yale in particular. My interviewer there pointed in one direction and said, "The library's over there"; another direction, "The laboratories are over there"; another direction, "The hospital's over there." "You come here and you're basically on your own. There's not much in the way of tests or requirements. You graduate if you can pass the medical licensing exam at the end of your four years."

That sounded fantastic. How much better or more avant-garde could you get than that? Another person at Yale asked:

"What year are you planning to graduate Brown?"

"Next year, 1957."

"Well, they've taken a Negro student this year, so there's no use in your applying for next year. It's pretty much one every other year. Next year's out."

One every other year? I thought. Why in the world couldn't they make it one every year?

So, with Yale out, I found my way to Harvard, where the dean of admissions, Dr. Kendall Emerson, interviewed me. Strangely, he was also supposed to interview me for Stanford. The two schools had worked out some sort of reciprocal arrangement. The Harvard interview went extremely well. Dean Emerson and I seemed to hit it off immediately. When we were done, he said, "Now let's set up a time for the Stanford interview. Saturday, November twenty-fourth at one PM would be good for me. Is that all right?"

"Yes sir," I said, thinking, Damn, Saturday in the middle of the football season? Then I saw the twinkle in his eye. One PM on November 24 was the kickoff time for the annual Harvard-Brown game. He had looked it up. "If you have some trouble clearing that date," he said with a smile, "we might possibly be able to work something else out." I left his office encouraged and hopeful. I didn't think the dean would have felt comfortable teasing me if he weren't positive about my chances.

When the letter came from Harvard, though, it was a disappointment. I was on the waiting list. So apparently Dean Emerson hadn't been that positive after all. A few days later the letter came from Stanford, a thick envelope, but I still opened it practically shaking with trepidation. And there it was—I was accepted! And with a full scholarship! I felt like I was floating. What didn't I feel? I was overwhelmed. I thought of Mom and all she had sacrificed, I thought of all the hard work, that it had all been worth it. But mainly I was overcome with happiness and humility and desire. I was going to be the best damned doctor I could possibly be. Absolutely the best! Nothing was going to stop me.

AFTER GRADUATION I WENT BACK to Memphis, looking forward to relaxing with my family and old friends, but also eagerly looking forward to September when I'd go out to Stanford as a first-year medical student—which I could still hardly believe. I had a job waiting for me in Memphis, the same one I'd had the previous three summers, lifeguarding at the city's Orange Mound Public Swimming Pool for Colored People.

That was a great job. The pool didn't open until 10:30, so I could sleep late. And other than occasionally pulling a little kid out of the water and being a bit of a policeman, there wasn't much to do but sit up on my high lifeguard's chair, talk with friends, and survey the Memphis belles, whose hair styles rarely allowed them to actually go into the water, but who didn't mind showing off in their bathing suits for appreciative eyes.

But that summer my head was full of thoughts about Brown, about the ideas and knowledge and intellects I'd been exposed to for the past four years, about the speeches I'd heard at the honorary societies I belonged to and at commencement from professors and visiting luminaries about scholarship and learning and being a student for life. And I thought, you know, you cannot just sit here on your behind at this pool anymore. You've got to do something more worthwhile with yourself.

So I started asking around, and it turned out that a new hospital had just been built in Memphis, the E. H. Crump Hospital, named after Boss Crump, who had died several years earlier after having ruled Memphis for what seemed a long lifetime. The E. H. Crump Hospital was for Negroes, though it was staffed almost entirely by white doctors and nurses. I had been accepted to medical school, so that seemed like the right place to apply for a job, and my mom and others I knew managed to make a connection for me, I think through Lieutenant Lee, who was still a political force in the city.

However that might have happened, word did get to the hospital and they decided to make a job for me. But they had to look around to figure out what a person like me could actually do, someone who had been a successful enough premed student but had no experience at all of medicine or patient care. What could I do? Well, they decided, I could be a "surgical technician," that is, a scrub nurse. I could learn the basics of that on the job and lend a hand in the operating room. The head operating room nurse would be my superior and my teacher, Nurse Ophelia Rice.

Like most all the staff, Nurse Rice was white. She was also, I thought when I met her, a little on the stern side. Nurse Rice was young, only twenty-seven or twenty-eight, and attractive—rumor was she had dated Elvis Presley. But she did not smile, at least not at me. That could have been because I had just been dumped on her to train, on top of her other responsibilities. But whatever it was, I got the sense that while she was going to handle this extra burden professionally, she was not going to do it with any great warmth.

Now I, unfortunately, was coming to Nurse Rice with a bit of an attitude myself. I had just turned twenty-one, which meant, among other things, that I was not a boy any longer; I was a man. And not only a man, a college man, who would soon be starting medical school. And since I was now a man, I was not going to be "Gus," or "Augustus," most especially not down here in the midst of this segregation. I was going to be "Mr. White." Just as Mom was always "Mrs. White" and Addie "Mrs. Jones."

But Nurse Rice started right off calling me "Augustus." "Augustus, do this" and "Augustus, do that."

"Excuse me," I said. "I'm a man now. So I'd prefer that you not call me by my first name. I'm happy to call you Miss Rice, and my name is Mister White."

That got no response at all, just a barely audible noise of some sort, not exactly a "humph," but something like it. But she obviously thought about it, because after that, although she refused to call me "Mr. White," she didn't call me "Augustus" either. Instead I was just "White." As in "White, take these sponges." Or more often just "Take these sponges." Consequently, I didn't call her "Miss Rice," but just "Rice."

That didn't make for a close relationship, but to her credit Ophelia Rice still taught me to be a scrub nurse. How to put my gown on, how to scrub my hands, what's sterile, what's not, how to drape a patient, what the instruments are, how to try to anticipate when the doctor will need which, how to pop them into the surgeons' hands the way they liked. Nurse Rice did teach me these things, and she taught me well.

Almost none of that would have been necessary, though, because my first day at E. H Crump Hospital was also very nearly my last day. Nurse Rice had introduced herself, handed me a cap and mask, showed me the men's locker room, and told me to go into Operating Room Three to observe a bit, just to see what it was like. She had something else to do, but she would be back shortly to look in on me.

Now, I had set foot in a hospital only once or twice since I was a kid, so I wasn't exactly used to hospital scenes. But I put the hat and mask on, as I was told, and stepped confidently through the doors of Operating Room Three. There, on the table in front of me, was a partially draped patient. He was lying on his side, and his bared back was painted in the middle with iodine. A doctor was leaning over him inserting a needle into his spine. The needle was about halfway in; it looked to be about a foot and a half long. I assumed the doctor was a surgeon, or maybe an anesthesiologist, and that he was administering some kind of spinal anesthesia. I stared at this procedure for about thirty seconds, the needle slowly entering deeper and deeper into the patient's painted back. Interesting, I thought. But suddenly I felt distinctly that I was about to faint. I had almost been knocked out once in college after being slammed into a wrestling mat. This was worse. A feeling of anxiety came over me. Nausea began welling up. The room started to wobble in front of my eyes.

I looked around. There were some signs and notices up on the wall. I'll be cool, I thought. I'll go over and read what they say, like I'm just orienting myself. That'll pull me out of this. So I walked over, as nonchalantly as I could, and started reading the sign. It was about cardiac arrest. But as I read, the sign began to rotate in a smooth, gentle, clockwise motion, slowly at first, then faster. Oh my God, I thought, I've got to get out of here. I'm going to faint. I can't faint. I've got to get out before I faint.

I walked out, my knees shaking, hoping nobody would see. I went back to the men's locker room, where I sat down, still nauseous, my heart thumping, sweating despite the chill of the air-conditioning. Oh shit, I thought, I can't be a doctor. I don't have it in me. I can't do it. I felt devastated, along with being sick. Oh, man, I thought, what am I going to do, what am I going to do? I don't know how long I sat there, ten minutes, twenty minutes, until finally I felt myself waking up, getting gradually back to normal, but still thinking, What am I going to do? I'm accepted to medical school, my father was a doctor, I've always wanted to be a doctor, everyone's expecting me. And now what? What in the world am I going to do?

Happily, nobody was in the locker room. And nobody had noticed in the operating room, or at least if they had, they hadn't followed me out. I took a deep breath. My head felt okay. The nausea was gone. And suddenly it came to me quite clearly. "You will now," I said to myself—I might even have said it out loud—"You will now get your black ass out of this chair and back into that operating room. Now!"

I walked down the hall and back to the operating room. Outside the door I took another deep breath and stood up as tall and strong as I could. I pushed open the door and walked in. On the table now the patient was all covered up. I could see the incision, though, and the surgeon working away through the incision. But it all seemed very objectified. I felt fine. I didn't turn a hair.

After that I was okay. I assisted on all sorts of operations that summer, some of them difficult and bloody, but none of them ever bothered me, at least not on that visceral level. Ophelia Rice and I never had more than a cool, impersonal relationship, but she was a competent nurse and a good teacher. And as I got better at my job, more familiar with the instruments and scrub procedures, I began to feel at home. The operating room was an exciting place. The surgeons all brought their personalities with them to their operations. Some were tense and curt with people, others relaxed and pleasant, as if it was the most natural thing in the world to be sectioning off someone's small intestine or cutting through a rib cage with what looked like garden shears. Some did their work with wonderful dexterity and grace, others were more plodding and awkward. But whoever was operating, the room was alive, there was always intense concentration, there was always drama and suspense. I was still pretty sure I wanted to be a psychiatrist—that's what I had been thinking all along at Brown. But surgery was obviously where the action was. I was going to have to take a good look at surgery.

I also saw that some surgeons cared about their patients more than others. Some of that was just personalities. One doctor might be warm and friendly, another might be colder and more remote. But sometimes the racial culture of the city intruded itself into the operating room. These were, after all, white doctors and nurses dealing with black patients. Eight years in the North had heightened my radar toward the biases that most Memphians considered a normal part of life, the condescension and patronization that characterized white attitudes toward blacks, white people's built-in sense of entitlement and superiority. I was usually pretty good at keeping an emotional distance from all that; I had had a lot of practice at it. But occasionally some incident would come crashing through my reserve. And one operation I saw left me enraged.

One of my good friends and early playmates from Memphis was a boy I'll call Eddie Dixon. He had sold newspapers with me when we were kids, and we were in school together until I left. Eddie's mom was a nice-looking lady about the same age as my mother. She had always treated me like one of the family when I was over playing with Eddie. I liked her a lot. And one day that summer Eddie got in touch with me to say that his mom was coming into the hospital. I told him I'd make it a point to see her, and then I noticed that her name was on the operating schedule. I was going to be her scrub nurse.

The next day Eddie's mom was wheeled in on the gurney, medicated but conscious and aware, though with all the people around she didn't notice me. She was obviously frightened, and she was shivering in the cold air of the operating room. I didn't know the operating surgeon; I had never seen him before. But his tone hit me immediately. "Get on that table, Janet," he said to her. "Be quick about it. We don't have all day." Then he went off to scrub. That was the kind of tone, brimming with disrespect and dismissal, that just set my teeth on edge.

While he was scrubbing, the anesthesiologist put Mrs. Dixon to sleep and intubated her. When we had her draped, the surgeon came back in and got started, making his first incision through the wall of the abdomen. From the operating room conversation beforehand, I knew that Mrs. Dixon had an extensive cancer of the uterus. There had even been some talk about whether the cancer was so involved it might be inoperable. But the surgeon had seemed kind of flip about it. I hadn't paid too much attention; all the surgeons had their personal styles. This one seemed irritated to have such a difficult case in front of him but at the same time casually cavalier about getting it done.

But as he got inside and got to work he immediately ran into problems. I could sense his frustration and anger growing. "Aw, damn," he said, "look at all that bleeding." Then to me, "Gimmee that Bovie, okay?" I handed him the Bovie, an electric scalpel that cauterized while it cut. "Look at this," he said, "there's even more damned tumor down here than we thought."

The more he uncovered, the more aggravated he got. All of which was making me extremely uncomfortable. But he kept going, and as he went on there was more and more blood flowing, pooling in Mrs. Dixon's interior cavities and bloodying the drapes. I didn't know exactly what was happening, of course, but a few years later when I was doing my own surgery rotation, Dr. Victor Richards, one of the true giants of American surgery, used to have a favorite line. "What is it, young doctors," he would say, "that is the unconscious patient's only defense against the incompetent surgeon?" And the answer was: "Hemorrhage."

I hadn't been exposed to Dr. Richards yet, but there I was, staring at an example of bleeding everywhere and the incompetent surgeon unable to control it. Hemorrhaging is a defense because the surgeon may give up and get out. But this surgeon just kept going. He was having a time. I didn't need to be a medical student to know that. I wasn't sure what I was looking at in there, but I could make out the uterus and a dark red amorphous bloody something or other that seemed to be the object of his attention. It wasn't till I was in medical school that I learned about the often vascular nature of cancerous tissue, how it can be friable and ooze blood when it's disturbed even slightly. Then I didn't know. But I knew a bloodbath when I saw one. Everything was bleeding and this surgeon was frustrated and angry. But he kept going, cutting and cursing, cutting and cursing, trying to do the surgery.

At some point, though, Mrs. Dixon's blood pressure started dropping precipitously and the anesthesiologist said, "She's in shock." The surgeon had them start pumping in a transfusion, but it didn't help. Then he just gave the whole thing up. I watched Mrs. Dixon die in front of me on the operating table.

I was in shock myself, seeing death right there in front of me for the first time. I felt a cold, explosive anger welling up toward this surgeon, who didn't seem to care much, or at all. "Okay," he said, "that's it. Damn, that was difficult. Let's get her out of here."

Usually when I assisted at an operation I tried to learn something, maybe about basic anatomy or what instruments were used for, or about surgical technique. But as this operation went on I had been thinking less about surgery and more and more about race. Here was this white surgeon treating his black patient the way he had, without respect, without according her the slightest shred of human dignity. And then to let her just die there, palled in her own blood? I was thinking about race the way black people in the South thought about race in 1957, with anger and resentment and a conviction that we should not be treated this way, that it was simply not tolerable.

I don't think it had quite hit me at that point that I was on the verge of entering a profession where white doctors treating black patients was the rule, and that there were a host of often hidden emotions and attitudes associated with that. It certainly had not hit me—because I didn't know yet—that, although at Brown I had been a member of a small but supportive minority group, at Stanford I was going to be a minority group all by myself. I hadn't given a thought to how I might fit in there. Nor to how I might get along afterward, in a profession where there were extremely few mainstream black doctors and almost no black university doctors who might be able to help ease my way.

3

BECOMING A DOCTOR: STANFORD

If you can fill the unforgiving minute
With sixty seconds' worth of distance run,
Yours is the Earth and everything that's in it,
And—which is more—you'll be a Man, my son!

—Rudyard Kipling

IT WAS PARTLY THAT OPERATION, the shocking
and dreadful nature of it, that had me thinking about more than
medicine as I drove out to California for my first semester at Stanford. Back at Brown, my experience with the DU fraternity had given
me a taste of what it was like to be up on the racial ramparts. As it
turned out, my ride out to Stanford also got me thinking more
about how maybe I could do something to help the cause, that is,
to help "advance the race," as the expression was.

The ride did that because I drove a brand-new Buick that belonged to a Miss Jackson, someone a friend had put me in touch with.
Miss Jackson was a few years older than I, and she also needed to get
to California. Our arrangement was that I would do the driving and
she would pick up all the expenses. Miss Jackson was on her way to
take a faculty position on the West Coast. She was one of the first
African American women to earn a higher degree in mathematics.

It was great to have her to talk to on the long trip, and beyond
great that she was paying for the whole thing. But much more important, she gave me a feeling of pride—I mean pride for who she was
and what she had done. She had proved something major. A black
person could be a high achiever in mathematics. If she could do it,

that meant that any black person might have the potential for something similar. Here was another proof to the world that we were as capable as anyone else, that we were not to be looked down upon. It sounds dated and somewhat naïve to be saying something like that nowadays. But then, African American "firsts" meant more than I can tell you. And somewhere in the mix of emotions about starting medical school, I was thinking—What about me? What can I do?

Stanford itself was a revelation. Just the look of the place was enough to knock you out. We drove up to the school through the famous Palm Drive, a colonnade of palm trees that created a rich green tunnel-like corridor that directed your eyes to a gigantic, sparkling, many-colored mosaic of gods, saints, men, and women. The landscaping, the architecture, the whole aspect of the place dazzled me. I had never been to Disneyland, but I had seen pictures. Stanford looked like some kind of fantasyland university. And the people, the students strolling around in this surrealistic setting, looked like they had been made for it. They seemed tanned, handsome, sculptured; they even carried themselves differently, more casually and confidently. And for some reason it seemed to me that a good percentage of these beautiful people were coeds. I'm not saying that my dedication to medicine was in jeopardy, but I did feel more than a momentary distraction. Or maybe it was just disorientation. Brown wasn't like this. And Memphis might have been on a different planet altogether.

Maybe that was partly because among all those students I did not see one single black face. Some time later I met Dr. Carlton Goodlet, a physician, civil rights pioneer, and publisher of the *San Francisco Sun-Reporter,* the region's black newspaper. Dr. Goodlet told me that I was the first African American student Stanford Medical School had ever had. I soon discovered that my matriculation at the medical school made me one of exactly four students of color on the campus. My three colleagues included a Samoan football player, an African American law student from Los Angeles, and a stunningly beautiful African American female graduate student in mechanical engineering who had, coincidentally, gone to Northfield School for

Girls, Mt. Hermon's sister institution. Not only that, this sister, Carole Coleman, had even appeared in *Jet* magazine; I had read about her. I saw her tooling around in her white MG sports car and I could not wait to make her acquaintance.

Whatever kind of social life I imagined for myself, though, got bumped into second place when classes started—which I guess is true for most first- and second-year medical students. But as demanding as the work was, my sixty-plus classmates and I (only four of whom were women) were kept at a high level of enthusiasm by the faculty, who seemed almost without exception brilliant, vastly knowledgeable, and invested in teaching us.

Probably the most popular was Walter Greulich, an eminent anatomist who was famous for having developed a method of radiological analysis that facilitated the identification of abnormal growth patterns in children. Greulich was originally from Germany and he had a strong Germanic aspect to him. For his lectures he wore a starched, sparkling white, crisply pressed lab coat. When he spoke he stood erect at the podium as if he were at attention. Then he'd begin striding around like a Prussian officer. But beneath the severe façade was a warm-hearted man, passionately engaged with his subject matter and possessed of an earthy sense of humor.

Given his stern presence, Greulich's humor had a disarming quality. During one lecture he described a feature of mammalian anatomy that is present in all male mammals other than those of the equids, marsupials, lagomorphs, and man—namely the baculum, otherwise known as the os penis, a penile bone that in the walrus, as Greulich mentioned in passing, can achieve a length of almost three feet. In the histology lab afterward, a number of us were discussing the whys and wherefores of this distinctly mammalian structure when Dr. Greulich came up, cleared his throat, and said, "Gentlemen, do I not detect the slightest tone of envy in this conversation?"

Underneath the starched appearance, Greulich had a streak of fun. He was also a deeply sympathetic person, someone you could talk to, which I did when I found myself having some trouble in the first-year biochemistry course. Greulich wasn't a biochemist, but he was a wonderful counselor and adviser. He took a true personal interest. He was on the admissions committee, he told me, and he remembered my application well. He not only had great confidence in my ability to get through my biochemistry problems, he had high expectations for me generally. Then he said, "Gus, do you know Dr. Montague Cobb?"

"No sir, I don't."

"Well, make a note of this. Dr. Cobb is a person you should make an effort to get in touch with. Dr. Cobb is a good friend of mine and a distinguished professor of anatomy at Howard University. It'll be good for you to get to know him. Tell him you're a student here with us and that I encouraged the contact."

That "Howard University" was the key. Dr. Greulich was telling me that Dr. Montague Cobb was African American. He knew that I would come across few if any African American role models or even teachers in my medical education. Other than at Howard and Meharry, there more or less weren't any. And he believed, rightly as it turned out, that Montague Cobb would be an inspirational figure for me. That was the kind of sensitivity Dr. Walter Greulich had.

Of course, I was, in a way, integrating Stanford Medical School, and it's likely that at least some of the faculty knew that and kept themselves aware of my progress. I never noticed any signs of it, though. As far as the racial atmosphere went, Stanford was as neutral as you could get, which I was especially grateful for given what my old friend Alvin Crawford was going through back in Tennessee.

Alvin Crawford lived right across the street from a great-aunt of mine in Memphis. I had known him and his family forever. Alvin had gone off to medical school himself, at Meharry, and of course he knew I was also in medical school. When I visited my great-aunt on my first vacation home, she said, "Oh, Alvin wants to talk to you. About medical school."

So I walked across the street and there he was. Sitting in his living room, he told me the story. The University of Tennessee College of Medicine had, of course, always been a whites-only institution. But now a consortium of education officials and Memphis political figures had decided it was time to integrate. They had asked Alvin if he would agree to transfer and become the school's first black student. What did I think?

I thought Yes. What an opportunity to knock down a barrier. The first African American at UT would have to have great strength of character as well as outstanding academic ability, and nobody was more qualified than Alvin. Alvin had made a reputation for himself in Memphis as a star student as far back as his school days, which was why they had come to him. No one wanted to take any chances on having this effort fail.

Apparently others gave Alvin the same advice I did, all of which fit in with Alvin's own inclinations, so he transferred. But integrating UT was not the same as integrating Stanford. When Alvin arrived he had already finished a semester's worth of courses at Meharry, including anatomy. But the Tennessee people decided that maybe the Meharry course was not up to their standards, and they told him he would have to take anatomy again. He did that, and received an honors-level grade for it. But, no, they told him, even though his grade was at the highest level, he didn't qualify for honors because, after all, this was the second time he had taken the course.

The reception in town was equally conflicted. Alvin's father was the longtime maître d' at the all-white Memphis Country Club. Some of the members knew about his gifted son and made it a point to inquire from time to time how he was getting along in his studies.

"How's your son doing?" they'd ask.

"Very well, sir. Thank you. He's in medical school now, at Meharry."

"That's good," said one doctor member. "I want you to give my *Gray's Anatomy* to your boy."

"That's excellent," said another doctor. "Let me give you one of my old textbooks. I'm sure he could make good use of it."

But when Alvin transferred to Tennessee it made quite a noise in Memphis. The city had been such a hard-line Jim Crow bastion for so long that breaking the University color line put a lot of people on edge.

"You know that *Gray's Anatomy* I gave your boy?" the first doc said to Alvin's father (as Alvin told me later). "Well, ahem, I think I'll need to get that back. My classmates . . . you know."

A couple of days later the second doctor said, "Listen, that book I gave you, that textbook? Your boy can keep the book. But here's what I want you to do. I want you to get that book and make sure you scratch my name out of it. Scratch that out completely."

In terms of its racial atmosphere, Palo Alto couldn't have been farther from Memphis. Unlike Alvin, all I really had to worry about was learning to be a doctor from people like Walter Greulich.

Another of Stanford's star professors was Victor Richards. Richards was widely acknowledged as one of the leading general surgeons in the country. His lectures were remarkable for their insight, thoroughness, and masterful organization. It's little or no exaggeration to say that they could have been transcribed verbatim and published directly. Amazingly, he delivered these impeccably detailed lectures without notes.

I studied under Richards at Stanford. Later he was my supervisor at the Stanford Lane Hospital where I did a year's surgical residency. Richards had been a student of Emile Holman, a preeminent surgeon at Stanford who had himself been a student of the great William Osler and an assistant to the father of modern surgery, William Halsted. Aphorisms were one of Richards's favorite teaching tools, as they had been for Osler and Halsted. Halsted had famously said (famously in the world of surgeons) that "hemorrhage is the only weapon with which the unconscious patient can retaliate upon the incompetent surgeon"; that is to say, by dying, which would illuminate the surgeon's shortcomings. Richards changed that to "Hemorrhage is the only defense of the unconscious patient against the incompetent surgeon." Namely, the surgeon may give up and get out before he actually does kill the patient.

In fact, Halsted's approach to controlling blood loss created a fundamental revolution in the world of surgery, a revolution that was epitomized by his student Holman and Holman's student Richards. Prior to Halsted, German surgical practice was the international standard, and German surgeons were famous for their daring and speed. The idea was to get in, do the surgery, and get out as fast as possible. One result was that operations tended to be enormously bloody. One turn-of-the-century English surgeon who toured the German clinics said that "German surgeons approach an operation on the canine principle of savage attack."[1]

Halsted's approach was exactly the opposite. He emphasized extreme carefulness and the absolute limitation of blood loss. When Halsted's precepts established themselves, they made possible the development of modern techniques in every type of surgery that requires precision, that is, more or less every type of surgery. In the process, American surgery came to the forefront. Victor Richards was in the direct line of this heritage. "Let thought precede action," he used to say. That is, make sure you know precisely what you are doing before you do it and be prepared to deal with any possible bleeding that may result.

As a medical student I understood that Richards was a master. Later, when I became a surgeon myself, I recognized that being his student made his heritage mine as well. And when I became a professor, I taught my own students to claim the heritage, especially significant, I thought, for black and other minority students to know that they, though they might be the first in their communities to enter the field, were equally heirs of the great Osler and Halsted as were their mainstream classmates, and that they should seize the meaning and pride of that heritage.

VICTOR RICHARDS was such a powerful, inspirational figure that he moved my own inclinations farther along toward surgery and away from my old idea of wanting to be a psychiatrist. That had started back in the Crump Hospital operating room, where I had been excited by all the action. The process got accelerated in my second year at Stanford when I was given a psychiatric clerkship and assigned a patient.

This patient was a middle-aged, schizophrenic, African American woman. My job was to introduce myself, talk to her, and try to get a feel for her illness. The patient was assigned to me randomly, but I was happy to start off with an African American. I had the idea that I would perhaps have a better understanding and be more empathetic toward black patients than a white doctor might be. But black or white, I couldn't wait to get started. Working with an actual patient—this is what I wanted; this is what I was so eagerly looking forward to. She was pointed out to me sitting on a bench in the sun. I couldn't get over there fast enough.

I sat down and introduced myself. "Miss Jones, how are you today? I'm Mr. White. I'm a medical student. I'm here to get to know you a little." My heart and soul were in this. I had learned all that psychology at Brown, I had picked up more in the clerkship. It was all right there. "How *are* you, Miss Jones?"

Miss Jones did not respond. Her face was a blank. She said not a word. She seemed not to have even noticed my smiling, enthusiastic presence. I might have been talking to a wall. Oh my goodness, I thought. This is not for me.

What a difference from the drama of the Crump operating room. Look at these doctors, I used to think while I was a scrub nurse there. They *do* things. They walk in, and when they leave they've fixed something. They took something out that shouldn't have been there, or they fixed something that needed fixing. Then they closed up and walked away. What a satisfaction must that be!

By my second year at Stanford I understood myself well enough to know that I really did want action, that I needed to feel I was accomplishing something tangible, something visible. And psychiatry, especially before drug therapies became widespread, provided very little of that.

That feeling for action was why, the moment I completed my Introduction to Clinical Medicine course, I put on a white coat and got myself down to the San Francisco County Hospital emergency room to help out, which Stanford allowed you to do at that stage of your training. San Francisco County mainly treated the city's poor and indigent. The patients were a cross section of humanity: black, white, Asian, straight, and gay. In the emergency room there, things came at you with machine gun rapidity. Fast, furious, and dramatic. Exactly the kind of situations that TV producers picked up on later for shows like *ER* and *Grey's Anatomy*.

County's emergency patients were a cross section, but a San Francisco cross section. The city was home to a large number of motorcycle riders, Hells Angels–type outlaws, and others. Bikers arrived with broken bones, internal injuries, and terrible head traumas. Then there were the ill and wounded from the city's gay community. San Francisco probably had the densest concentration of gays and lesbians in the country. Even before AIDS there was plenty of disease, also victims of violence: gay lovers who had been assaulted by their rough partners. Some of these involved long-term couples; the County Hospital residents casually referred to them as "married," as if that was something completely normal. That was a revelation to me. I knew about gay sex, of course. But married gay people? I'd never heard of such a thing.

San Francisco also had a reputation as a big drinking place. At one point it was famous for having the most bars per capita of any city in the country. One of the first patients I saw come in was a disoriented Caucasian male vomiting blood. The ER docs and the attendings knew what it was immediately—advanced alcoholism with severe liver cirrhosis. They sometimes handled three of these a day.

They jumped in, working to stem the bleeding. Cirrhosis occludes the main vein draining the liver, causing blood to back up into the esophageal veins, which become distended and can rupture. Once that happens there's hell to pay, which was what I was now witnessing. The docs got a transfusion in to try to keep up with the bleeding. Then they fought to get tubes down the man's nose and the back of his throat, past the pharynx and the lungs, so they could pump up a balloon and compress the ruptured vein, hoping to close down the tear. These days there are more advanced methods. Today's surgeons are often able to go down endoscopically, place clips or bands around the veins, and suppress the bleeding that way. But in 1958 those techniques were still in the future.

I mainly watched, helping with anything I could, which was very little. The doctors fought heroically to stop the hemorrhaging, but after six or seven hours of doing everything they could think of, the man went into shock and died.

That was my first day. After that I just couldn't get enough. I'd be down there whenever I could, sometimes two or three nights running. I was so excited I didn't even want to sleep. I'm sure my contributions, such as they were, diminished exponentially, but I was there. I started IVs, I moved people from one table to another, I took histories. I was able to bandage well, so I bandaged. If they needed a pint of blood or the result of a test, I ran to the laboratory to get it. I was as up for this as I could possibly get. I was flailing away, jumping from one thing to another, totally involved. Then I'd go home and sleep the sleep of the dead so I could get back to my normal medical school pace.

So, I had this firsthand experience with real action at County Hospital. I had the distinguished Dr. Victor Richards as a teacher. And I had another, equally memorable, teacher who became one of my personal icons of medicine, this one an orthopedic surgeon.

Dr. Don King was six foot three, lean and erect. His steely blue eyes peered out from behind horn-rimmed glasses. His face was usually lit by a broad smile. He strutted around the wards making rounds, just short of a caricature, almost like a frustrated actor, exuding pride and confidence. But the smile gave him away. He might have been an actor, but he was an immensely likable actor. He was also a gifted surgeon, and an extraordinary teacher.

Don King's pedagogical specialty was clinical patient presentation. Western medical history credits the great French neurologist Charcot with epitomizing this teaching technique. Charcot was long before my time, but I can't imagine his presentations were more effective than Don King's. Here's my memory, for example, of how he presented a patient with a recurrent dislocating patella of the right knee—a highly effective presentation, since half a century later I can still precisely envisage the entire episode.

There's Dr. King strutting back and forth behind his lectern, and there's the patient, a twenty-eight-year-old Caucasian male wearing only a pair of brief bathing trunks, half sitting, half reclining on a stretcher in front of the lectern. The amphitheater is full of students.

"Today, boys and girls," intones Dr. King, "you will learn about the orthopedic entity of the recurrent dislocating patella. First, let me describe for you the relevant anatomy of the knee . . . ," at which point Dr. King launches into a detailed description of the kneecap, or patella, its attachment to the quadriceps muscle above and the patella ligament below, the groove of the femur that allows it to glide up and down, and the various other associated structures. Dr. King shows all these on a diagram as he talks, then comes around to the patient and moves his right knee up and down. We watch the patella move as Dr. King bends and straightens the patient's knee, though we cannot see the femoral groove upon which the kneecap glides so smoothly.

"Now, boys and girls," he says, "notice how the normal patella moves easily, without any pain whatsoever. And now, here is the dislocating patella. *See!*" His scream almost knocks us out of our seats, as with his two thumbs he pushes the patella from the inside toward the outside of the knee, out of its groove, dislocating it and locking it in place off to the side of the knee. It's the patient now who's screaming—in agony—flexing forward and backward and writhing on the table while Dr. King strides purposely around him and, with his right hand, pops the patella back into its normal position. The patient suddenly relaxes and emits a long sigh of relief. Every student in the amphitheater does the same.

We speculated among ourselves after this and other dramatic presentations whether Dr. King might be administering an analgesic beforehand, and possibly even giving some drama lessons to the patients to maximize the impact. We never discovered if he did or didn't. But each student in that class retained an exact knowledge of the patella, its attendant structures, its normal and abnormal movements, and how to treat it if it dislocates. We were still talking about that at our forty-fifth class reunion.

I loved these demonstrations. I loved the action of the ER and the OR. I seemed to naturally gravitate to the surgeons, especially to Dr. King. After that second year I knew surgery was for me. And of the various surgical subspecialties, I was most drawn to orthopedics. The fix-it sensation, the satisfaction of accomplishment when you've made something right, is epitomized by orthopedic surgery probably better than any other specialty. Most often, orthopedic patients have problems that are fixable. You screw something back together, or rebuild it, or strengthen it. You make your patient's life better in some obvious way that leaves him or her happy with the outcome and gives you a sense of fulfillment as a physician.

Because I was convinced I wanted to be an orthopedic surgeon, and also because my mother had recently remarried and moved to Cleveland, Ohio, I began looking to see if I could get some kind of summer position at the Case Western Reserve University School of Medicine orthopedics department. I carefully composed a letter to Professor Charles Herndon, a prominent orthopedic surgeon who was chief of the department there. I was a junior medical student at Stanford, I told him, interested in a career in orthopedics. Might there possibly be any summer research work I could do?

I did not say in this letter that I was a Negro medical student. I was extremely conscious of having left that out. In this letter I was not African American. I was not the first African American at Stanford. I was—"a medical student." Period. Inquiring about a summer job.

A short time later I received a reply from Dr. Paul Curtis, a distinguished orthopedist and research scientist at Case Western. Dr. Herndon had passed my letter to him. Dr. Curtis informed me that he did have a research project I could help with. There was a stipend attached. Here were the articles I should read to prepare myself. When could I start?

This was excellent news. But as the summer approached, a thought started preying on my mind. After all, I had not been totally honest in my initial letter, had I? Well, yes, I had been honest, just not totally candid—not mentioning my race. Suppose Professor Curtis did not like black folks, certainly a possibility. Suppose Professor Curtis assumed that I had been morally obligated to let him know who I was so that he could have rejected me out of hand or at least met with me to assure himself I was qualified or that I wasn't going to be unruly and cause disruptions. Who knew what kind of racial thinking might be going on in Professor Curtis's mind? Would he think I had consciously deceived him? I didn't even know if Case Western Reserve University School of Medicine had ever had a black student. I assumed they hadn't. And if they hadn't, why not? I mean, even Stanford had never had a black student before.

As I arrived in Cleveland to report to Professor Curtis, I decided I would have to test him. I would give him "the flickering eye test," which I had just thought up. I would walk into his office, shake hands, and say, "Hello, Dr. Curtis. I'm Augustus White." And while I was doing this I would look straight into his eyeballs. If his eyes flickered, I'd have to consider that Dr. Curtis harbored some autonomic, or maybe even overt, racial feeling and that he might well consider that he had been duped. I wasn't sure what I would do if that were the case, but it would most certainly make a difference.

In Dr. Curtis's office, I did exactly that. We shook hands and I looked directly into his eyes and introduced myself. Dr. Curtis's eyes did not flicker even for a single instant. I was home free. I felt as if I had won the lottery.

I didn't know how lucky I was to have made Dr. Paul Curtis's acquaintance. First, he was an excellent teacher and research director. Second, the research itself—on the degree to which systemically administered antibiotics enter the synovial fluid of the joints—was significant. Third, and far more important to me personally, was that he turned out to be a superb mentor and was probably *the* instrumental person in helping me further my education in orthopedics and, consequently, my career.

This last started with a conversation I had that summer with a good friend and tennis-playing partner named Bobbie Dibble. Bobbie was three or four years my senior. He had done his medical training at Howard Medical School. Now he was an internal medicine resident at Cleveland City Hospital. Everyone in the educated black community knew who he was and knew he was destined for great things.

After a tennis game one afternoon, Bobbie and I were talking about our careers and I told him I was going to be an orthopedic surgeon. There was a long pause. Then Bobbie said, "What do you mean, you're going to be an orthopedic surgeon?"

"Well," I said, "you know. I'm going to finish up school, get a residency, complete my training. The usual."

"I see," he said. "And where do you think you'll get this residency?"

"I don't know yet. I'll apply."

"Gus," Bobbie said, "do you know how difficult it is to get an orthopedic residency? Do you know of any black person who's an orthopedic surgeon?"

Now that I thought of it, I didn't.

"So, what makes you think *you* can get a residency?"

"Well, I'll apply."

"Gus." Bobby sounded tired, as if he were explaining something that shouldn't need to be explained. "Gus, I think there's probably two, maybe three black orthopedic surgeons in the entire country—at Howard and at Harlem Hospital. That's it. You can't just apply anywhere. There's no point. You have to ask around, see what kind of possibilities there might be. You're working here at Case, right? Ask them. Maybe they'd give you something."

So I did ask. I went to Dr. Curtis, explained my desire to be an orthopedic surgeon, and asked his advice about a residency. What about Case, for example?

Dr. Curtis, whom I knew well by this time, and who, I knew, liked me and liked my work, did not answer directly except to mention that Dr. Herndon, the chief, was a southerner. Thinking back, it's more than likely that Dr. Curtis would have wanted me as a resident, so I wouldn't be at all surprised if he had already felt Dr. Herndon out on the subject. "Gus," he said, "I'll be very happy to help you look for a residency." Then, very tactfully but very clearly, he told me that I could not apply for a residency the same way I had applied for my summer job; I could not leave out the fact that I was Negro. If I did that I'd be spinning my wheels and letting myself in for considerable frustration. People would, of course, find out, and a lot of departments would not consider me a viable candidate. "It's unfortunate," he said, "but that's the way it is."

"But," he also said, "I'll help you navigate this. Why don't you give me a list of places you're interested in. I'll help you amend that to include places where I know people. Then I'll make some calls about you."

Which is what happened. The result was that together with Dr. Curtis I selected eight or nine places that seemed particularly attractive: Yale, the Hospital for Special Surgery, the Mayo Clinic, Harvard, the University of Michigan, Columbia Presbyterian, and several others.

At the end of that summer I made the rounds of all the institutions that had invited me to interview. The standard practice for medical students is that when they finish their four years of medical school, they are matched through a national program with an institution where they will do a one-year internship, sometimes in their desired specialty but more often in a general internship, which gives them experience in a number of specialties. The internship further trains young doctors and prepares them either for a general practice or for the extended, specialized training of a residency at the best institution they can get into.

I hit the road in my old Plymouth, eager to see the famous schools and hospitals I was applying to. I thought I'd probably like all of them. Whether they were going to like me was another question. Dr. Curtis had friends in some of these orthopedic departments, but not all. I assumed that few if any had fielded many, or even any, black candidates before. Bobbie Dibble had said that other than at Howard and at Harlem Hospital there were virtually no African

American orthopedic surgeons. Starting out on this trip I was brimful of enthusiasm and confidence, not to mention curiosity. But somewhere in my head a small voice was also asking if I really knew what I was getting into here.

Some of my interviews put that question out of my mind. When I arrived at the Mayo Clinic's main pavilion I was greeted by a uniformed gentleman at the reception desk. When I told him I had come for an interview, he said, "Of course, Dr. White. Welcome to the Mayo Clinic." I knew that Dr. Curtis was friends with Mayo's chief of orthopedics, Dr. Edward Henderson, who made it clear toward the end of our talk that they were interested in me and encouraged me to seriously consider training with them. Other interviews went less well. Several were so ice-cold I felt as if I had brought a chill wind in with me. No one I talked with ever mentioned race, even subtly, but with one or two eminent chiefs, I couldn't help but wonder.

Probably the place I was most interested in was Yale. I had been so impressed by their medical school four years earlier, but then they'd had that unfortunate one-Negro-every-second-year admissions policy. This was four years further on, though, and back then I had been just another anonymous college student looking at schools. This time around I'd be dealing with people on a more personal basis, most especially because of Dr. Curtis's introduction to his colleagues.

When I started laying out my plans for this big interview trip I had called my old DU brother, roommate, and close friend John McDaniels. John and his wife, Beverly, lived in New Haven, where John was a law student at Yale. John and I had been through a lot together in college, including that aborted national Delta Upsilon convention—John was supposed to have been my co-delegate to that. I had also been the one who originally introduced John and Beverly, so I felt a small but definite level of personal involvement in their marriage. My Yale interview would give the three of us a chance to visit and catch up.

"What exactly are you going to be doing here, Gus?" asked John, when we sat down in his living room.

"Well, I'm applying for a job. I'm trying to get a place as an intern or resident at Yale–New Haven Hospital."

"No kidding," said John, then yelled out into the kitchen: "Bev, hon, isn't Gus Lindskog at the Medical School?"

I knew who Gus Lindskog was. Everyone who knew anything about surgery did. Gustaf Lindskog was Yale's chief of surgery, as near to a divinity as a surgeon could be.

"Beverly, why don't you call him up and see what he's doing?"

So Beverly dialed up Yale's chief of surgery. "He's free," she called from the kitchen. "He's just sitting around the fireplace having a cup of coffee."

"Bev, ask him if we can come out and say hello."

"Yes, he says it's fine, we should come on out."

It turned out that John had been in the Navy with Gustaf Lindskog's son, and when John was accepted at Yale Law School the son had told him to look up his parents, which John did. Professor Lindskog and his wife had helped John and Beverly get settled. They had been friends ever since.

I understood something about the value of contacts, but whoever expected anything like this? A half hour later I was sitting in Professor Gustaf Lindskog's living room listening to Beverly and John tell him what a fine person they thought I was and what a positive contribution I would make to whatever program I was part of.

That get-together could not have harmed my interview the next day with Wayne Southwick, Yale's orthopedics chief and Dr. Curtis's good friend. Dr. Wayne Southwick was like a breath of fresh air, especially after one or two of the less-than-cordial interviews I had been through. I felt so comfortable with him that I asked directly, "Dr. Southwick, do you think I have a chance at a position here, I mean, as a black person?"

"Without a doubt," he said. "The only thing we're interested in is getting the absolute best people we can."

The University of Michigan was another good experience. Dr. Curtis had called his friend and colleague there, Dr. Robert Bailey, a rising star in the world of cervical spine surgery. I found out later that Dr. Bailey had a reputation for tough love, with the major accent on tough. But he greeted me warmly and seemed interested in me. Then he took me over to meet Michigan's renowned chief of orthopedics, Professor Carl Badgley. Professor Badgley's interview was more like a long, relaxed talk. It didn't hurt either that Don King, my orthopedics mentor at Stanford, had been Professor Badgley's student. King followed up my interview with a strong letter of support, so I had good hopes that something positive might happen there too.

When the medical student/internship matches were announced that spring, Michigan turned out to be the top institution on my list that had also chosen me. I was excited about that; Michigan had one of the country's best programs. An internship at Michigan also meant I'd have an excellent chance at a follow-on orthopedic residency. I had good hopes too that, even though Mayo or Yale hadn't selected me for an internship, the positive interviews I'd had in those places and at some others might give me a step up in applying to their residency programs. My future, thanks to Bobbie Dibble and Dr. Curtis, seemed to be looking pretty bright.

The Stanford graduation ceremony that May was quite wonderful. I had been elected president of the medical school student body, so I got to give a student address—and this in front of my mother and Aunt Addie (Doc had, unfortunately, died a couple of years earlier). My uncle Arnett White from Chicago was also there; he was my father's younger brother who had been so supportive of me my entire life. My San Francisco girlfriend of two-plus years, Kathy Phalen, attended as well, which was an additional pleasure. My mother tried not to be too effusive—she had always kept a tight rein on any tendency I might have toward getting a big head. But even she couldn't hide her pride. I wondered too if maybe she wasn't thinking about my dad as well. He had died sixteen years earlier, and now here I was, his son, a doctor now myself.

AFTER THE CEREMONY I drove Mom, Addie, and Uncle Arnett to the airport, then packed up for my own long drive to Memphis, which I needed to do as expeditiously as possible so that I could make the wedding of an old roommate from Mt. Hermon, Bill Holmes, to Clarice Dibble, Bobbie Dibble's sister. They had asked me to be one of the groomsmen. I had exactly seventy-two hours to get to Memphis, then to Tuskegee, where the wedding was going to be.

I was going to make this trip in my brand-new black Chevrolet convertible, which Addie had helped me finance as a graduation present. I had actually just picked this car up from the dealer. It was so new that I had a temporary paper license plate for it instead of the regular plate, which the registry was going to mail to me. Like all new cars in those days, the Chevrolet required a break-in period. I wouldn't be able to drive it more than fifty miles an hour for the first 500 miles. That was going to put a crimp in my timing. On the other hand, I was taking two other medical students with me, so with three drivers we'd be able to keep going nonstop. My apartment mate, Doug Warner had graduated with me and needed to get to a summer job in Florida. His friend Jeffrey, another med student, was coming with him. We figured we'd only stop for fuel and bathroom breaks and to buy food, which we'd eat in the car. The rest of the time one or another of us would be behind the wheel, one would be navigating and making sure the driver stayed awake, and the third would be catching some sleep in the backseat. Then, every four or five hours we'd rotate. This would maximize our speed. With any luck, I'd make it to the wedding with a few hours to spare.

For most of the trip our plan worked to perfection. We swung down to Southern California, then headed out toward the famous Route 66, rolling eastward with the top down, the wind in our hair, and the radio blaring out rock and roll. The trunk was packed tight with our clothes and books. Our gas money stash was in the glove compartment. The sun was hot, but a semicool breeze washed over the car, especially after we passed the 500-mile mark and could lean on the gas pedal. None of us wore a shirt; the warmth was just too delicious. I was especially pleased to find my skin color darkening to what I considered a more satisfactory tone, which complemented my ten-gallon, Jimi Hendrix–style Afro nicely.

Our schedule was tight, but we were keeping to it. I was sure I was going to make the wedding on time. As we were getting toward Little Rock, Arkansas, Doug was driving, Jeff was riding shotgun, and I was sleeping soundly in the backseat after a long stint behind the wheel. But somewhere west of town something happened. The first I was aware of it was when a deep southern backwoods voice intruded into my sleep. "Baw, you come over heah whal we check out this vehicle. Both you baws."

The car had stopped. I came out of my sleep slowly and realized that we had been pulled over by police. Doug and Jeff were getting out. The police apparently hadn't seen me yet. They had pulled over what they thought were two white boys—maybe they had been speeding, maybe it was the paper license; I didn't know. Whatever it was, though, it wasn't a racial stop.

"You baws jes stand over theah, lemme see your license." And at that moment I raised up out of the backseat, Jimi Hendrix Afro and all. "Whoa!" said one cop. The second just looked startled. Two white boys, now all of a sudden a black one too. I was wide awake now. I just knew what they were thinking. White boys and a black boy driving around together in a brand-new Chevrolet automobile; something ain't right here. "You jes stand over heah too," the older cop said. "Roy, you search the car"—this to the younger one.

"Hey George," said the junior guy, poking around in the glove compartment. "They got money in the glove box! Damn, there's whiskey in here too!"

There was—a mostly full pint bottle I had bought for a BYOB graduation party commencement night. I didn't drink, and nobody else at the party had bothered much with it either, so I had taken it along. This was going from bad to worse. White guys, a black guy, money—our gas stash—whiskey.

"You baws got any weapons in this vehicle?"

"No, sir." "No, officer." This from Doug and Jeff. I hadn't told them about the snub-nosed .38 under the front seat. I had been driving back and forth across country alone for the past four years. Who knew what might happen out in the middle of nowhere if I had a flat tire, or at some truck stop if I stopped for gas? The .38 gave me a certain feeling of comfort, probably false comfort, but anyway, there it was. I didn't say anything; I just closed my eyes and hoped Roy wouldn't find it.

Then, "George! C'mere, George. Lookit!" And Roy held up the gun, which I had inherited from my stepfather. He checked the cylinder. "And it's loaded!"

"You baws stand theah and don't move," said George. "Roy, you call the criminal investigator. Tell him what we got an' tell him to get hisself down heah."

We stood there. We all stood there. Time passed. The criminal investigator didn't come. I wasn't sure if I still had a wedding in my future. For some reason, though, I wasn't afraid, which I probably should have been, which any southern black man with an ounce of sense should have been. But, I kept thinking, I'm a medical student, actually, I'm a doctor. All this is silly; we didn't do anything wrong here.

So finally I said to the senior policeman, "Look, officer, we're good citizens. We're all medical students. We just graduated from medical school. We've got our textbooks in the trunk, you can check them. They've got our names in them so you can see that it's the same names as on our licenses. I have the paper license because I just bought the car out in California where we were in school. They give you a temporary license plate there before they send you a permanent one. Please, you've got no reason to keep us here."

Apparently this had an effect, besides which, I think the cops were getting tired of standing around in the sun waiting for the criminal investigator to show up. Finally the senior one figured there really wasn't anything going on, and that there wasn't any point in drawing this out. "Y'all can go," he said, and he gave me back the envelope with our gas money. The junior one had the gun. He looked at the senior one, then he looked at me, then back at his partner. Then he gave the gun to the senior cop. The senior looked at me, looked at the gun, looked at me again, obviously running this dilemma through in his head. Then he gave me the gun.

"Thank you," I said. "Now, what about my whiskey?"

"Baw," he said, "if you don't get out of here . . . ! You must be crazy!"

We got into the car and left. Quickly. I hadn't been trying to be a wiseacre—it was my whiskey, not theirs. But within a couple of minutes I started thinking that we could not only have found ourselves in jail, we could have found ourselves under the jail. And then I started thinking that if we had been three black guys, that's just where we probably *would* have found ourselves. More than likely.

4

BECOMING A SURGEON: YALE

I had discovered the weight of white people in the world.

—James Baldwin

I CAN'T IMAGINE what I was thinking, asking for my whiskey back from those Arkansas cops. Could four years in laid-back California have partly dulled my racism antennae? I didn't think so, but maybe it had.

Not that Stanford had been completely without incident. The core of the fourth-year curriculum there was what was called the medical/surgical clerkship. In this program, medical students were assigned patients whom we would follow for a semester. We were responsible for meeting them, getting to know them, doing physicals, taking histories, doing full workups, and presenting our patients and their cases to the attending physicians. Our grade in this clerkship was crucial, by far the most important of any of our medical school grades. In a very real sense it told you how well (or not so well) you were progressing at this stage of your work toward becoming a doctor. I badly wanted to do well.

It wasn't that the medical students hadn't met and worked with patients before this, but previously it had been mainly as on-lookers. We offered our observations, we learned how experienced doctors perceived and evaluated symptoms, our knowledge base was tested and expanded. But this was the first time we had been given any personal responsibility. It was a little nerve-racking. I would say that everybody, myself included, was pretty much up to speed in terms of the medical understanding expected of fourth-year students. But the personal side of it—that was something else entirely. How do you, the doctor (actually, the not-quite-a-doctor), talk to a patient effectively, establish rapport, demonstrate empathy, convey confidence, develop a relationship? This is a test of your human skills, which will be so important to you once you're truly out in the clinical world.

I naturally liked to meet and talk to people, so I thought I might do pretty well at this, and my first encounters did go well, even if there were one or two challenges. Balancing the scientific, objective side with the subjective, personal side was something I felt comfortable with. But even seasoned clinicians face surprises sometimes. My surprise was Mr. Jameson.

Mr. Jameson was in serious trouble. In his fifties, he had been referred to Stanford Hospital from Washington, D.C., with a severe case of lymphoma. His situation was dire, but not yet terminal. He was facing a long, very difficult time, and he was trying to adjust to his diagnosis.

We had made rounds on him that day with a full team: the resident, the attending, the medical students. In the evening I was rounding again, this time by myself, looking in on the three or four patients I had been assigned as part of my clerkship. Given his situation, I figured Mr. Jameson could use a little special attention. He had no family nearby and few if any visitors. I thought I'd try to give him some support. Be sympathetic, upbeat. Cheer him up some, if I could. Let him know that, in me at least, he had a friend as well as a doctor.

I walked into his room and said hello. I reminded him that I was his student doctor; I was just dropping by to ask how he was feeling and to talk a little. We began to chat, making small talk, trying to find some areas of mutual interest. I felt we were striking up a nice rapport.

"I notice you're from Washington," I said. "That's an interesting place. So many things to see and do there."

Mr. Jameson perked right up. I thought, Good, the man wants to talk about his home town. Excellent that he's not completely overwhelmed by his illness.

"Yes," he said. "Washington's an interesting place, all right. Very interesting. Except for one thing."

"What's that, Mr. Jameson?"

"Too many niggers." He paused and shook his head. "Just too many damned niggers."

I almost laughed out loud. Then I felt my anger rising. Goddammit! I thought. Here I am trying to cheer this bastard up. I didn't confront him, but I'm sure he could see I wasn't enthused by his remark. "Well, Mr. Jameson, I'm going to say good-bye now." I don't think he knew I was African American—my light complexion again. So it wasn't a direct, in-your-face insult. It was worse. One white guy expressing himself candidly to someone he thought was another white guy. Expressing his own true feelings, and expecting, of course, that those feelings would be shared.

So, what to expect at Michigan, where I was headed after the summer, where I'd be immersed in the world of doctor-patient relationships? A place where I'd be the first black doctor most of the other docs and patients had ever dealt with. I do want to say first, though, that three or four days into my summer vacation I got a postcard with my grade for the medical/surgical clerkship. It was an A. The fact that I remember that so vividly indicates how important it was to me. I had given up church long before this, but I was so grateful for that A that I actually dropped to my knees and said a little thanksgiving prayer. I felt like Stanford had just given me its blessing for what I had chosen as my life's work.

The University of Michigan Medical Center was not a place where you could break in slowly and gently. I had lucked out in getting this internship. Michigan was one of the top places in the country, and the slot they had for me was what was called a "rotating surgical internship," which meant six months rotating among surgical specialties and six months rotating through other departments. This kind of internship wasn't around generally, and it didn't stay around very long either. But there it was, and it was perfect for me. Whether I was perfect for it, though, was another question.

That was a question I couldn't have answered during my first weeks at Michigan—in spite of all my preparation, my dedication, all my hope and desire to become a surgeon. The pace during those first weeks was so mind-numbing, so dizzying, that I thought maybe I just wasn't cut out for this after all. I was paired up with a junior resident, Dave Kline, who later became a renowned neurosurgeon. Dave quickly became my teacher, my mentor, my friend, and a source of inspiration. But even with his attention and support there were moments during those first weeks when I thought I might just go under.

Our ward there had forty or so patients—all of them our responsibility. The operating room went full throttle, all day long. Dave and I alternated, switching off days in the ward and in the OR. I'd get started every morning at six or six thirty and often find myself still working at nine or ten. I got little sleep, especially when I was on call. My head was swimming all the time. I even thought back once or twice to my introduction to the OR at Crump Hospital in Memphis, when I had almost just given up. I wondered if maybe I hadn't made a huge mistake, thinking I had what it takes to be a surgeon.

I had a hard time, and it gave me more than a little anxiety, though in fact there was nothing unusual about what I was going through. My experience wasn't different from that of most new surgery interns. And what I eventually found is that it's like being in training for football or wrestling. You muscle up for it, you develop the strength and stamina and inure yourself to the hardship. The work conditions you, and after a few weeks you find, a little to your surprise, that you're not going to die after all. Working like a crazed obsessive gets to feel more or less normal.

But getting conditioned to the hours and stress was just the beginning of a learning process that was full of challenges and interesting situations. Years later, when I began teaching at Harvard, the esteemed Derek Bok was president. His wife, the philosopher and ethicist Sissela Bok, had written a scholarly book on lying in which she argued, among other things, that small lies, "white lies," can be as unethical as bigger lies. Not true always, of course. And certainly not true in the case of Ed Veralnik, an eighteen-year-old boy who was one of Dave's and my patients, an eighteen-year-old boy on the verge of death.

Ed Veralnik was dying from a fairly rare gastrointestinal condition called pseudomembranous enterocolitis. For some reason, which we could not immediately determine, his intestinal bacteria had gone badly out of balance. Normally, the various intestinal bacteria coexist in the gut by keeping each other in check. But if the level of competition somehow gets thrown out of kilter, one group might take over, with potentially dire consequences for their mutual host, in this case, Ed.

In Ed's gut much of the normal bacteria population had been reduced to almost nothing. As a result, one strain, c. difficile, was running amok. Ed's c. difficile were killing him—wreaking havoc with his fluid and electrolyte balance, obstructing his ability to absorb nutrition, building up toxins in his bloodstream. There was one last-resort strategy to counter this cascade of damage: replenish Ed's normal background bacteria; that is, infuse them into his gastrointestinal system. The only question was: How?

Unfortunately, there's no such thing as an intestinal bacteria tablet or therapeutic fluid. These bacteria have to be obtained from the environment. They exist pretty much everywhere, but in microscopic quantities. There is, in fact, only one place where normal intestinal bacteria congregate in high concentrations, which I, frankly, had never given any thought to. As George Zuidema (the attending physician), Dave Kline, and I moved away from Ed's bedside after examining him, Zuidema said, "Gus, please develop a bacteria cocktail for this young man and administer it this evening."

"Sure," I said, not having the vaguest idea where I was supposed to get such a cocktail.

As soon as Zuidema moved off, I collared Dave, my resident and friend. "Dave, an intestinal bacteria cocktail? Where in the world am I supposed to get an intestinal bacteria cocktail?"

"Well," said Dave. "When was the last time you, uh, moved your bowels?"

I will leave the reader to visualize the next scene, which took place with the aid of a basin, a spoon, a saline solution, and a lavage bag.

When I had prepared the cocktail, I went up to Ed's room, leaving the lavage bag at the nurses' station while I went to talk to him, knowing I was about to commit the sin of skirting the truth.

"I know you understand," I said, "that your problem comes from the absence of certain bacteria that normally exist in your intestines. What we have to do to try to heal you is replace those bacteria. We'll do it through a thin tube I'll insert through your nose and down the back of your throat into your stomach. I'll help you with that; passing the tube won't be difficult. Then I'll infuse the therapeutic solution. Does that sound okay to you?"

"Sure, doc," said Ed, a very pleasant, polite young man. "Sounds fine."

Once we got the tube down, it took almost an hour to administer the "therapeutic solution." Which sounded fine to Ed, but he might have had more than a little trouble with it had his doctor been more candid. But the treatment did, in fact, put him on the road to recovery.

That bacteria cocktail was a challenge of one kind. A couple of months into my internship I handled my first surgery, which was a more relevant, and more instructive, challenge.

By that time Dave thought that I was ready to take on a small surgical procedure by myself. He asked if I would like to do it—to check out my confidence level—and when I told him I would, he went off to assist in the operating room, leaving me alone to excise a small scalp tumor from one of our patients.

The tumor was about the size of a large olive, just under the patient's skin. We had judged that it was noncancerous and that removing it shouldn't present any special difficulties. I could do the procedure in a little treatment room that was just off the ward.

I asked one of the nurses to get the patient, a Mr. Alexander, set up and prepared, and while she did I went over the procedure in my head. I'd scrub up, put on my cap, mask, and gloves, adroitly and expeditiously anesthetize the area, incise the skin, dissect out the tumor with either a scalpel or a small dissecting scissors, close the skin, bandage the wound, receive Mr. Alexander's heartfelt thanks and the nurse's congratulations on my first surgery, say a satisfied good-bye, and get back to my morning rounds. Mission accomplished. No muss, no fuss.

In the treatment room the nurse, a competent but recent graduate of the Michigan nursing school, had Mr. Alexander prepped and comfortably positioned. Hair shaved, area cleansed, sterile instruments laid out and organized, syringes and local anesthesia ready to go.

I anesthetized the area quickly and professionally. I made a bold, definitive incision over the central part of the tumor. Victor Richards and Don King had never been tentative in their initial incisions, and neither was I. Now to evert the skin over both sides of the tumor and begin the dissection, hemostats ready to control any bleeding.

But suddenly my nice clean incision was awash in blood. How could I not have known? The scalp bleeds. It bleeds like hell. I was totally unprepared for the innumerable, tiny vessels that profusely and seemingly irresistibly gushed forth with blood. I put in my hemostats to clamp them off. But the thick, fibrous tissue that constitutes a large part of the scalp made it difficult to place them effectively. I put pressure on the bleeders, which closed them down, but the moment I removed the pressure they started right up again. I should have had a Bovie, the electric cauterizing knife, prepared for this. But it was too late for that now.

With the nurse helping to apply pressure, I forged ahead with the dissection, worrying about the blood loss, which wasn't life threatening but was a lot more than it should have been. I wondered if Mr. Alexander was getting anxious, listening to my quiet requests for more sponges and more instruments, wondering whether this very young doctor and even younger nurse really knew what they were doing.

With a lot of sweat, a lot of sponges, and a lot of hemostats, we finally got it done. The blood stopped coursing. I excised the tumor. I closed and bandaged the wound. As we had judged, the tumor turned out to be benign. There were no complications. From an objective point of view, my first operation was a success. From my point of view, it was a tense, instructive lesson that had me talking to myself for days about what it means for a surgeon to be totally prepared and what can happen when he or she is not.

IN 1961 JAMES FARMER started the freedom rides. Groups of black and white volunteers rode Greyhound and Trailways buses into the South to test discrimination in terminal waiting rooms, restaurants, and restrooms. In some places the riders were beaten by mobs, in others they were arrested. The Ku Klux Klan followed the buses, inciting violence wherever they could. Robert Kennedy sent U.S. marshals. Protests were going on in Mississippi, Alabama, and elsewhere. Martin Luther King launched a regionwide voting drive. The civil rights movement was ramping up. Excitement was in the air. Anger and determination were in the air. And me? I was sitting on the sidelines, doing nothing. Of course, I was working fourteen-hour days at the University of Michigan Medical Center, which was hardly nothing. But what was I doing "for the race?"

"Doing something for the race" was an expression I had heard since childhood. When I was growing up, "doing something for the race" could have meant doing something big or doing something little. Joe Louis and Jackie Robinson did big things. Mr. J. A Hayes, the principal at Manassas High School, did something little when he asked the visiting white supervisors to please remove their hats, they were in a school. That might have been a small thing, but not in the students' eyes it wasn't. Not in those segregated, subservient, suppressive times. What Mr. Hayes did took guts. Doing something for the race meant standing up and being counted in whatever way you could, like Mom and Aunt Addie demanding respect from store clerks. It meant standing up and insisting on your human dignity.

I had a short-lived career as an activist before I went off to Mt. Hermon, when I was eleven or twelve. I had decided at some point that I could get people to go out and vote. I must have heard someone talking about voter registration and how colored people had to get themselves registered. How that was reasonable and right, how we were equal and how we had to exercise our rights. So I started going around to people's houses, telling them how important a thing that was for them to do. Some people were actually polite. "Well," they'd say, "I'm not sure. I'll think about it." More often I'd hear, "Boy, you get on out of here. I ain't going to do no voting. Think I'm goin' down there and get myself beat up?"

So, that didn't work out too well. Later when I would come home from Mt. Hermon for vacation I'd go to my grandmother's church where they'd ask me to give a speech. They wanted something inspiring, something along the lines of, I've made it, all of us can make it. That was doing something for the race too.

But here I was in Michigan, age twenty-five, and the country was in turmoil. A whole social revolution was gathering steam, and I was sitting on the sidelines. I didn't feel good about that at all. Underneath my immersion in my studies, the frustration of it gnawed on me.

I'm not positive how that might have worked out, except that before I left for my internship, Bobbie Dibble had told me that once I got to Michigan I should make sure to look up Dr. Reuben Kahn. Dr. Kahn was a good friend of Bobbie's father, who was a distinguished physician in Tuskegee, Alabama. According to Bobbie, Reuben Kahn was a person I could trust, someone who would be happy to lend a sympathetic ear to a young black intern, should that intern ever need it.

Dr. Reuben Leon Kahn was a famous man. When I met him he was in his mid-seventies but still working hard as a senior professor and scientist at the Michigan Medical Center. Dr. Kahn was an immunologist. He had developed the standardized test for syphilis and had done other landmark work in serology. He had a gentle, grandfatherly way about him, and Bobbie was right, he was sympathetic, someone I found it easy to talk to. Not only that, he seemed to take a liking to me personally, and he made me understand that he was interested in me and my career.

One night Dr. Kahn invited me to dinner and at some point the conversation turned to civil rights and racial issues, as conversations almost inevitably did in those days. I don't think I said anything overt about how I was feeling, but I did talk about my huge admiration for Martin Luther King and the others who were doing such earth-shaking things. I think Dr. Kahn sensed my frustration at not being able to take an active role in these events that obviously meant so much to me, "the cause," as I'm sure I put it.

"Gus," he said, in a soft, even loving, tone, "please allow me to give you some advice. I think your job right now is to focus on your medical education and on becoming the best, most effective doctor you can possibly be. You can't do that and also be a civil rights leader, or a demonstrator or a revolutionary. It doesn't work like that. Right now you need to develop your knowledge and your professionalism. Once you've done that, once you establish your credibility, you'll find yourself in a position of recognition and influence. That's when you'll be able to have some real effect. That's the time you'll be able to make moves that will really count."

Maybe Dr. Kahn told me what I wanted to hear, soothing the guilt I was feeling. Be that as it may, his words seemed to make all the sense in the world. They comforted me. They reinforced my desire and determination to keep on with what I was doing.

The usual progression for an apprentice surgeon is to move through an internship into a one-year general surgery residency and from there to either continue with general surgery or find a residency in a subspecialty: cardiovascular surgery or neurosurgery or one of the others—in my case, orthopedic surgery.

As far as my general surgery residency went, I knew what I wanted. I wanted to go back to Stanford and work under Victor Richards and Don King, both of whom had made such a powerful impression on me in medical school. I couldn't have been happier when I was accepted at the old Stanford Lane Hospital, soon to be renamed Presbyterian Medical Center now that the medical school had moved into a new hospital facility in Palo Alto. A contingent of senior doctors had remained on staff, though, including Richards, King, and several other internationally known surgeons.

My year at Presbyterian was everything I anticipated. Practicing surgery under Victor Richards steeped me further in the Halsted ethos of meticulous preparation and minimal blood loss. With Don King and his colleagues, I got to work with some of the world's most renowned orthopedic specialists, practicing my own skills under their guidance and gaining confidence almost daily.

Along with my work at Presbyterian, I started volunteering as a prison doc at San Quentin in Marin County outside of San Francisco. One of the hospital orthopedists was "Curly" Watson—"Curly" in deference to his completely bald pate—and Curly Watson handled orthopedic treatment at the prison, doing procedures that could be performed under local or regional anesthesia, lots of knee and foot surgery especially.

Every other Saturday I made my way out to San Quentin to lend a hand. Going into that place was a reality check. I'd walk in and the gates would clang shut behind me, slamming out the normal life of San Francisco with its jazz clubs and restaurants and the colorful Beat Generation street life and communal feeling of those years. It was a sound that always gave me a chill, a harsh announcement that I'd entered a different, menacing world.

Treating prisoners, though, wasn't different from treating other patients, except not always. I was drawing blood once, having a little trouble getting a needle in—the man seemed to have no visible veins—when another patient piped up, "Here, let me help you, doc. Let me do it." And bam, he slid it right in. Like a magician. Some of the prisoners were upbeat and friendly, making me think about how irrepressible people can be, whatever their circumstances. Others were sullen and uncommunicative, and I'd often wonder what crimes they might have committed.

The scrub nurses were a special case. They were all convicts, but some were as good as well-trained nurses outside. I saw their humaneness and compassion, the way they cared for their patients—whatever the scrub nurses might have done that put them there. As bad as that might have been, in the ward and in the treatment rooms their humanity was on display every day.

That was one side. But San Quentin showed you the other side too. Over time I understood that the ward was a dangerous place. Not for the doctors, but for the patients who were assigned beds there, too ill to go back to their cells or recovering from operations. If you had enemies, the ward was an easy place to die. It didn't happen that often, but it did happen.

Sometime during the latter part of the year I received a letter from Yale University that I had been accepted as an orthopedic resident. It wasn't a complete surprise. Dr. Southwick had been extremely encouraging during my interview there, and Gus Lindskog, Yale's chief of surgery, had informed me while I was still at Michigan that a second-year resident's slot had opened up, and that he thought I'd be able to manage it even though it would mean skipping a year. I hadn't taken up his offer. I was extremely eager to go back to Stanford to study under Dr. Richards and Dr. King. But even if it wasn't a surprise, Yale's acceptance was still great news.

As I prepared to go off to New Haven, in the back of my mind was the fact that I had been told not to apply to medical school there because of their one-Negro-every-other-year policy. We were six years farther along now, and a residency was far different from a medical school application. But the issue of race had hardly gone away. I had seen the letter of recommendation Michigan's chief of surgery had written to Dr. Lindskog. I had apparently lived up to Michigan's expectations. Then at the bottom in a handwritten scrawl, one chief to another, he wrote: "I imagine you've noticed that this is a pale, colored boy."

When I had interviewed two years earlier with Dr. Wayne Southwick, Yale's chief of orthopedics, he had said he didn't care if I was colored or what. He was just looking for the best students he could get. Back then I had had some good interviews and some bad ones, but good or bad, none of the other eight or nine chiefs I talked to ever actually mentioned race, whatever they might have been thinking. The issue was too delicate to bring up overtly. But Wayne Southwick wasn't a delicate person. Southwick had grown up on a Nebraska farm; he was the kind of man who did what he thought was right and let the chips fall where they may. I was going to be the first black surgical resident at Yale, but he hardy even considered that.

Many years afterward I asked him, "Did you expect some blow-back when you decided to admit me?"

"Yes," he said. "And I got some. But I thought, that's their problem, not mine."

Southwick's opposition came from the heads of Yale–New Haven Hospital and Newington Children's Hospital, two places where Yale residents trained and helped carry the load. Neither had had a black resident before, and it seemed that neither was all that eager to have one now. Despite Dr. Southwick's lack of regard for the "problem," word had apparently gotten around.

Wayne Southwick, as I was to learn, was well known for the way he selected his residents. Yale, being Yale, could have its pick of applicants. But he had his own criteria. Since everyone had the grades and recommendations, he looked for people who had different backgrounds and varied interests, but who he thought could work as a team. By different backgrounds, he didn't mean diversity in the way we think of it now—he came to Yale from Johns Hopkins in the late 1950s, long before diversity became a national focus. But even then he was aware.

"Being from Nebraska," he told me, "my wife and I had had very little contact with black people. But when we came to Johns Hopkins we saw separate drinking fountains and separate eating facilities. Baltimore was segregated back then. We were shocked. The hospital even had white and colored blood banks. Which, by the way, I never paid any attention to. If someone came in needing a trans-fusion I gave them whatever was available."[1] I think Southwick got a kick out of the idea of some segregationist running around Baltimore with a pint or two of black blood in him.

Wayne Southwick had a reputation as one of the country's top cervical spine surgeons. I knew that. I also quickly learned that his residents loved him, as I came to do also. He was an extraordinary mentor. He was a gentleman, but didn't mind a fight either, which he had his share of, in particular with the surgery department, which controlled the orthopedics budget and had administrative jurisdiction. Dr. Lindskog was an ally of his. But when Lindskog retired, Southwick and the new chief of surgery were regularly at loggerheads. Southwick was carving out increasing autonomy for orthopedics, and that exacerbated the natural clash of cultures between the two types of surgeons, general surgery tending to be hierarchical and unforgiving while orthopedics is by and large more easy-going and peer friendly (this is, of course, an orthopedist's opinion).

Southwick's office was in the basement of Silliman Hall, with a window at ground level. If Southwick didn't want to see the surgery chief when he came over, he'd climb out the window and bicycle off. Things got so heated that the surgery chief fired him. Of course he couldn't fire him from his professorship, just from his chairman's job. Southwick more or less ignored him and stayed on doing the work. Tellingly, none of the candidates Yale contacted for the position agreed to take it. As one of them said, "You've got a perfectly good chief already. Why would I want to come in?" Southwick was eventually reinstated. Later the dean fired the surgery chairman.

If Wayne Southwick was against you, you'd have to hold on to your hat. If he was on your side, he was on your side. Period. I was thankful he was on my side, if only for the moral support, which I needed—not often, but sometimes.

In order to receive accreditation, orthopedics departments must include a certain amount of children's orthopedics in their training. Yale's residents trained at Newington Children's Hospital near Hartford. Newington was one of the county's highest-rated children's hospitals, and the surgical group that practiced there was happy to have Yale residents to help out in return for providing clinical experience and a level of formal instruction.

Most of this instruction took the form of meetings in which we residents would present the cases we were working up and caring for. These were full presentations. We would review the literature as it related to the pathology, discuss the diagnosis and treatment options, and make our recommendations. In the course of this, the hospital surgeons would quiz us on our understanding of the case, occasionally expressing their approbation, sometimes challenging our data or conclusions, and either approving or canceling our surgical plans—the main purpose of the exercise being instructional.

And most of the time it was instructional. But not always. The attending surgeons usually posed questions meant to explore and clarify. But there was more than a little one-upmanship too, attendings trying to embarrass the residents and show up their real or simply apparent shortcomings. That's certainly what I was feeling, from a couple of the attendings in particular. Their hostility was palpable; it was obvious they had a problem with me.

"Augustus, did you do a white [white blood cell] count on the patient?"

"Yes, of course."

"What was it?"

I told him.

"I see, and what about the differential counts?"

He was asking about the separate counts for the basophils, eosinophils, lymphocytes, monocytes, and neutrophils.

"I've got them right here in the chart, doctor."

"Oh, really? Not in your head, Augustus? And why is that?"

Bam! I gotcha, you sonofabitch. Maybe even I gotcha, you black sonofabitch. Not said, of course, but written in the gleeful look on his face.

"Augustus. A polio patient has weakness in the quadriceps muscle. Is it more difficult for him to walk up an incline or down?"

I'm thinking—is that in the literature? I don't think it is. Let's see, biomechanics of walking, no . . . gate analysis, no . . . damn. "Doctor, I'm not sure of the answer to that."

"Yes, we can all certainly see that."

Bam!

There was nothing I could do about any of this, but I did make it a point to wear a heaven-sent pin the National Urban League had just put out—a white button with a black equals sign on it. I put that on my white jacket where it stood out prominently and made me feel a lot better.

Now, I knew very well what was going on here. Or did I? Interns and residents do experience that kind of thing. These days the term they use for it is "pimping." An attending who does that to a student is pimping him or her. Doctors aren't necessarily angels. Some of them like to intimidate and harass subordinates. And when they do, the harassee gets to thinking: Why is this happening? Is this person just having a bad day, he got up on the wrong side of the bed? Or maybe he doesn't like me personally for some reason? What?

But for me there was an additional question: Is this really just personal? I mean, okay, he's got a right not to like me. Or is this character I'm dealing with here really a racist bigot? Like I think he is. An important question.

Important, but what a distraction. I have to sort through it. I ought to be focused like a laser on the medical issues, the facts, the analysis, the patient, the problem we're trying to solve. Not: Why did you do that? Not: Do I have to get into this with you? And if so, how?

Here's an entry from my journal during that period:

May 18, 1966

Paranoid level seems a bit high today. What I mean is that on service rounds, back over at our home hospital, I concentrated too much on the political considerations—that is, how other doctors were reacting to me, what they were thinking, were they with me or against me. This was very distracting, as I should have been focusing on thinking about the clinical information, interpreting it and expressing my views. Guess I'm mentioning this as a case in point of the extra baggage a black man has to juggle in these pioneering type environments. I talk to myself a lot. Not worried about that . . . yet.

For me, this was a running liability, as I think it is for many young black physicians. It drains energy. You have to decide, Do I retreat, do I retaliate, do I walk away? And you may or may not be happy with your decision. So then you find yourself thinking about that. And these thoughts running through your mind are not productive. The last thing you need is to be worrying about such things. I'm sure I've burned up some capital and goodwill from time to time in reacting—though, fortunately, not a lot. Some black males do burn up a lot.

As a young resident, I was at a disadvantage. I hadn't yet built the confidence I needed to handle this kind of problem. And it didn't help at all that there wasn't an older, wiser head to talk to—not a single black physician on staff at Newington, or Hartford Hospital, or Veterans, or Yale-New Haven. Nor a single black surgery professor at the medical school. Which made Wayne Southwick's support all that much more important. Not that I discussed these things with him then (though I did later), but I knew I could count on him 100 percent. If I got into trouble he would back me up, no ifs, ands, or buts. Most all of Wayne Southwick's residents thought of him during their training and throughout their professional lives as their father or their wise elder brother, myself very much included. I may have had more reason than most, whether he was aware of it or not.

Southwick had done his own residency at Johns Hopkins and was a faculty member there before coming to Yale. That meant that he, like Victor Richards, was in the direct William Stewart Halsted tradition of surgery. On the clinical side, Halsted had set a standard for meticulous surgery. On the pedagogical side, Halsted advocated and practiced the art of allowing trainees to learn through doing. That was the Hopkins system, that was Victor Richards's system at Stanford, and that was Wayne Southwick's system at Yale.

My first chief resident at Yale, though, hadn't gotten the message. Part of the chief resident's job is to guide and teach the younger staff, the residents and interns; to lead them through and give them experience with various surgical procedures. But the chief resident when I came in was, first, not a ready communicator—he talked extremely little—and second, he did the surgery himself, all of it, from open to close, in surgeons' terms "from skin to skin." He didn't give any of it away. And I was like a racehorse. I wanted to do everything and learn everything, as fast as possible. Faster. Let me make the incision, let me close the wound, let me do the procedures I can. Let me help out on the ones I can't.

I was a frustrated man. But I thought, Well, if I'm not learning from him because he's not talking, let me at least try to learn some other way. After that, I did my clinical work as expeditiously as possible, made myself available by page, and immersed myself in the radiology department teaching files, which housed a huge collection of X-rays relating to bone diseases and tumors of the musculoskeletal system, maybe eight or nine hundred of them, each file with an instructive explanatory note taped to the bottom. An incredible teaching tool. By the time I moved from the chief resident's service to another service—three months later—I had studied about 80 percent of the files, which was enormously helpful to me in understanding orthopedic pathology.

After that experience, the Southwick system of learning by doing kicked in for good and I could practically see my abilities improving week by week. I was doing what I had hoped and intended: I was mastering the skills that were going to make me an effective orthopedic surgeon. If I had been frustrated those first few months, now I was satisfied. More than satisfied, I felt alive. I was beginning to feel the joy of being able to do good surgical work.

I also began to gain more insight into the intimate connection between some back problems and emotional issues, particularly interesting to me given that earlier on I had been considering a career in psychiatry. The psychogenic origin of back problems is a difficult area. It can be awfully hard to tease out direct relationships. But there's no question that the phenomenon is very real. In one case

I dealt with as a resident, the relationship could not have been more straightforward, or more dramatic.

The patient was a thirty-three-year-old truck driver, a short, slight man who was grotesquely bent over at the waist and somewhat tilted to the left. He couldn't right himself at all; nor could anyone pull him up straight. But when he was lying on his back he straightened out as if there was nothing wrong—the salient sign that there is nothing wrong physically. The condition is called camptocormia, Greek for "bent body." It was first noted in certain soldiers during World War I.

According to the literature, camptocormia has no known physiological cause. We conducted our own extensive battery of tests, of course, but were unable to find any clinical evidence of a problem. Our patient's bone structure and musculature seemed completely normal. With all the tests negative, it seemed that the explanation very likely lay in the realm of the mind.

Working on that theory, we consulted with one of the staff psychiatrists, who got permission from the patient to conduct a pentathol interview. This is an unusual procedure; I doubt that even many psychiatrists have been involved in one. Sodium pentathol is a short-acting barbiturate that has the effect of relaxing a patient; in a certain dosage it induces coma and is often used as a precursor to administering general anesthesia. In smaller doses it lowers inhibitions and can make a subject readier to talk candidly to an interviewer (or interrogator; sodium pentathol used to be called the "truth serum," though its effectiveness for that end is questionable).

We had an anesthesiologist administer the drug; then the psychiatrist began a gentle questioning. How did the patient feel? A little sleepy? How was his health generally? When was the back condition worse? When was it not so bad? What did he do for a living?

"I'm a truck driver," he said.

"What kind of truck do you drive?"

"An eighteen-wheeler. I'm up there in my cab, I look down on everyone. I'm like the king of the road. But then I go home."

"Yes? You go home. What happens when you go home?"

"Then I come home and my wife treats me like I'm worthless. She puts me down. She looks down on me all the time. She makes me feel so small. She beats me right down. My back gets so sore and bent."

All the doctors in there—the anesthesiologist, the psychiatrist, the other resident, and I—were there as medical people, objective, scientific minded, professional. But we all felt terrible for this poor guy. No one expected anything so simple or so poignant. His wife beat him down, and his body bent under the blows, as if the psychological effect translated directly into the physical symptoms.

Camptocormia is rarely simple and often does not respond to psychotherapy. But this case did. The psychiatrist made recommendations for us, to help us positively reinforce our patient. The patient and his wife also began a course of family therapy, and over time his condition ameliorated significantly. Most psychogenic back pain is harder to treat and, while not so dramatic, can be equally real and sometimes equally debilitating too.

Our patient here was an object lesson for me in the complexities of back pain as I moved through my residency and began thinking about what my next step was going to be after Yale. Not surprisingly, Wayne Southwick had a lot to do with that, too.

One option was private practice. I could try to find a group to join, or even possibly go off on my own. Private practice was attractive in some ways. In a practice I would be concentrating on my patients without the necessity of doing research or teaching. I also wouldn't be beholden to layers of administration, department heads, deans, committees, and the uncertainties of academic politics. My success would be more determined by how good a surgeon I could be, the kind of reputation I could develop, rather than by circumstances and people beyond my control.

The other side was that I wasn't sure what group might be interested in having me. No one had offered me a job so far, and my experience with the orthopedic groups at Hartford and Newington had been less than wonderful. There was a real difference between the kind of welcome I had received from university professors and from private practice doctors. To a large degree, I thought that probably reflected the assumption of private practitioners that a black person wouldn't be acceptable in their practices. Other doctors might be unlikely to refer patients to a black orthopedist. That's what I thought. Of course, no one actually knew. This was 1966. Outside of Harlem Hospital and Howard there were essentially no black orthopedists in practice.

No doubt, going into private practice would be chancy. Meanwhile, Dr. Southwick was moving me in subtle and not so subtle ways toward academic medicine.

In addition to our clinical training, each resident was expected to do a research project that related to the Yale program. The assignment Southwick gave me was to conduct a follow-up study of patients who had undergone a certain spine operation called anterior cervical fusion. This operation was related to the Yale program in the sense that Dr. Southwick himself had helped develop the operation, and he and other Yale surgeons had performed many of them. But a follow-up study would have far more than parochial significance. The anterior cervical fusion operation had been a significant breakthrough in spine surgery, but no large-scale assessment of its effectiveness had ever been done. A paper on this subject would be of great interest to all orthopedic surgeons, especially to the rapidly developing contingent of spine surgeons.

Southwick's contribution to developing this operation had taken place while he was at Johns Hopkins. His professor there was Robert Robinson, chairman of the Hopkins orthopedic department and a world-renowned spine surgeon. Robinson, Southwick, and another Hopkins surgeon, George Smith, had found that it was more efficacious to operate on the upper segment of the spine (the cervical spine) by approaching it through the front of the neck rather than the back.

Most neurosurgeons and orthopedic surgeons had characteristically gone in through the back, which is intuitively the proper entry point, since the spine runs down the back. But the Robinson-Southwick-Smith contribution was clarifying that the anatomy of the neck area allowed for an easy entrance from the front through planes of fibrous tissue that could most often be parted by hand, without the use of a knife or scissors. Additionally, entering through these tissues kept the procedure away from vital nerve and vascular structures, making the operation safer as well as easier.

The follow-up study I undertook was labor intensive, to say the least. I reviewed all the charts for the sixty-five Yale–New Haven Hospital patients who had undergone the operation, recording twenty-plus indices for each operation on a flow chart. I reviewed X-rays for each, and interviewed and administered psychological screening tests. I had preliminary results ready to present at the Little Ortho-pedic Club conference, where Dr. Southwick introduced me. Completing the entire study took several more years, and I was joined in the work by Dr. Southwick and several other researchers. But in the end it was published in the *Journal of Bone and Joint Surgery* and was a frequently cited reference for a number of years.[2]

Wayne Southwick, of course, knew that this study would be important, and that as the lead author I would gain some recognition in the academic community especially. He also identified an area of orthopedics, somewhat underdeveloped in the United States, where he thought I could make a contribution. I might not have fully recognized the extent to which he was grooming me for aca-demic medicine—in my own mind I was still mulling my options—but that's what he was doing.

The field Southwick felt was inadequately developed, at Yale and elsewhere, was orthopedic biomechanics. Orthopedics deals with the interaction of the skeleton and muscles, orchestrated by the nerves. The entire structure acts as a machine that carries loads, protects stability, and enables movement. Biomechanics looks at machine aspects of the body generally. Orthopedic biomechanics deals with the machine aspects of the musculoskeletal system.

In New York City, up in the heart of Harlem on 125th Street, is the Hospital for Joint Diseases, one of the top orthopedic hospi-tals in the country. And it so happened that two medical scientists there, Victor Frankel, an orthopedist, and Al Bernstein, an engineer, were offering a training course in orthopedic biomechanics. So Southwick registered himself, me, and two other residents, and off we went to Harlem to study biomechanics. I liked to joke that my friends used to huddle up close to me as we walked along 125th, which I think they actually did. Not that there was ever any trouble, but up there at that time they did stand out.

Frankel and Bernstein had put together a truly effective course, which substantially benefited all of us. Along the way we learned that Frankel had studied in Sweden under Carl Hirsch, the great Gothenburg University professor who was regarded as the father of orthopedic biomechanics. And that gave Wayne Southwick an idea.

Why not, he thought, send me over to Sweden? If I learned biomechanics with Hirsch, I could come back to Yale as a junior faculty member. That way Southwick could kill two birds with one stone. First, he could remedy Yale's deficiency in the area. Second was an idea he had obviously been hatching for some time. "Gus," he said, "I really want you to consider academic medicine. As far as I'm concerned, you could be the first black medical professor in the Ivy League." The first time he mentioned that I thought he was being a little overenthusiastic. But after he said it a couple of more times, I knew he was serious.

5

COMBAT SURGEON:
DEATH AND OUR COMMON HUMANITY

It was a most terrible spectacle. I wish I could commit to paper the feelings with which I beheld it.

—Frederick Douglass

Like sitting at the delta of a river of blood—but you adjust and count days and are grateful that it isn't your blood.

—Memphis Slim

IN FACT, THERE WAS ONE black Ivy League medical faculty member already, Marvin Shelton at Columbia. But Southwick and I were not aware of that. There had also been at least one black Harvard professor in earlier times, William Augustus Hinton, who joined the medical school faculty in 1918. Neither of us knew that either. Not that Wayne Southwick's intentions would have changed, of course. His real purpose wasn't to make me a first of some sort, it was to get an African American person onto the faculty. He thought it would be good for Yale, good for the profession, and not least, good for the black community.

With those things in mind, Southwick began lining up an NIH grant that would get me to Sweden to study with Professor Carl Hirsch, the great biomechanics man. But before I would be able to do anything like that there was an obligation I had to take care of.

I finished my residency in June 1966. A year earlier the Johnson administration had sent combat troops into Vietnam. Now the war was going full blast, and physicians were subject to a special doctors' draft. I was young, I was single, I was an orthopedic surgeon. There wasn't an iota of doubt that I was going to go. I was so sure of it I had even made arrangements with my draft board. They agreed to let me finish my residency, then they'd take me.

I did have other options. I could have joined the National Guard. I could have gone into the Navy Reserve or the Public Health Service. But none of those seemed quite right. Here I was, fully trained, after so many years. I couldn't wait to get out on my own and be what I had worked so hard to be. And where in the world could I do that instantaneously at the highest volume in the most needed place other than Vietnam? Besides, I thought, I'm not going over to kill people; I'm going over to save them. And besides that, how about what I owed? I had grown up during World War II. As a kid I had watched all those newsreels and war movies. I had marched around the living room singing "Remember Pearl Harbor" as the song poured out of our radio. *Remember Pearl Harbor, as we fight for vic-tor-y. Remember Pearl Harbor*... Our soldiers had protected me then. Shouldn't I be giving something back?

The answer was: Yes. I was ready to jump over there and do what I could. I could go to Sweden afterward.

From my journal:

July 8, 1966

Fort Sam Houston Army Base, San Antonio, Texas

This is the basic training site for the U.S. Army Medical Corps. Here we learn to dress, salute, load and shoot a .45 caliber pistol and an M-16 automatic rifle. They put us in steel helmets and boots. Psychiatrists, internists, orthopedists. We learn to use a compass and crawl on our bellies. More important, we learn how to debride wounds.

Debriding wounds may be the most significant skill in the military surgeon's repertoire, and it's not one they teach in medical school.[1] The purpose of debriding is to cleanse a wound of all foreign material: dirt, bullets, metal fragments, feces—anything that might be in it. In the laboratory at Fort Sam Houston we studied the various types of wounds and what they do to the body. A high-velocity bullet, for instance, has a phenomenal amount of kinetic energy. If it hits bone it transmits so much energy that bone fragments in effect become additional bullets, wreaking havoc with any tissue or organ they hit.

In debridement you not only want to cleanse the wound of foreign material, you also want to cut out all the dead tissue. Dead tissue can cause as much pathology as dirt. Dead tissue serves as a nidus, a source of nourishment for organisms that can infect the wound. So, we studied dead tissue; we learned to recognize it: dead skin, dead subcutaneous tissue, dead fascia, dead muscle. We learned how to cut it out using Metzenbaums (surgical scissors curved at the end), erring always on the side of thoroughness, going after tissue that will soon be dead as well as tissue that has already died. After two weeks we were making judgment calls more easily, practicing on sheep. Soon enough we'd be applying our new skill on the bodies of American soldiers.

Another verse of that old marching song running around in my head went *Remember Pearl Harbor, as we do the Alamo.* Since Fort Sam Houston was in San Antonio, home of the Alamo, I decided I had to see it. The old mission and fort was one of the great patriotic sites, a place where American soldiers had fought and died for their country, similar to what was happening now. The likelihood of my dying in Vietnam wasn't great, but quite a few American soldiers were doing just that, and war was unpredictable. Who knew what might happen once I got over there?

From my journal:

July 8, 1966

Yesterday I went to the Alamo, in uniform, practically overflowing with patriotism. It should have been a tremendous source of inspiration. I read the names of all the heroes, the 100 or so that are engraved on bronze plaques inside the fort. Then I came to the final plaque. The very last entry read: John—Negro Boy.

I'm sorry, but this just ruined the whole damned thing for me. Was he really a boy? Or was he a Negro man? Who died as the others did, fighting for his country? Didn't he have a last name, like all the others? If he had a last name, didn't anybody know it? If he was really only a boy, what was he doing fighting to the death alongside men? Was his first name really John, or was it just known that there was some Nigra who got killed, so we'll just call him John? Should I be proud and thankful that they even bothered to mention him? Should I be proud that my race was represented at all in some positive way in a historic American event?

Or maybe I should ask myself, what kind of Tom would be there fighting in the first place. No . . . no. Can't ask that about him without asking the same thing about me, can I? Without bringing up all my rationalizing about being a doc and being needed and not killing but saving lives, which I never know how much is rationalization and how much is my honest belief.

In retrospect, I think maybe it was some of both: rationalization and honesty. Pretending to myself that I was just another American who ought to be doing and acting just like other ordinary Americans—and at the same time truly feeling that despite everything, at bottom I really was a legitimate part of America, and acting that way because it was true.

From my journal:

August 19, 1966

I just arrived in Vietnam. I am full of intense emotions, too complex to thoroughly explain. These include feelings of disgust, depression, determination, anxiety, frustration, hope, along with a certain romanticized sense of adventure. The country is hot, humid, dusty, dirty, and has the subdued but distinct smell of human waste.

The 85th Evac Hospital in Qui Nhon, where I was assigned, was the largest military hospital in Vietnam. Later they built another hospital in Qui Nhon that had actual buildings, but in 1966 the 85th Evac was a series of Quonset huts laid out end to end and connected by covered cement walkways. At the near end of the Quonset huts was a large helipad and parking area, which was where the helicopters and ambulances came in with their loads of wounded troopers.

Living quarters for the doctors and other officers consisted of a huddle of three-man tents a hundred yards or so from the hospital.

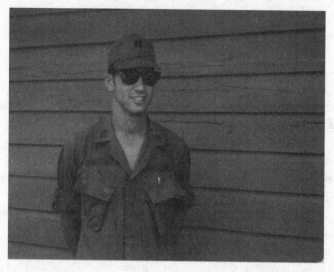

Captain, Medical Corps, United States Army, Commander 139th Medical Detachment K.B., Qui Nhon, Vietnam, 1966–1967. From the AA White Family Collection.

I plunked myself down in the one they showed me and stowed my duffle bag. With the cots and my tentmates' gear there was no room to move or do anything but lie down. Feeling a little gritty from the flight up to Qui Nhon, I went to take a shower. A cold-water shower, as it turned out, which left me shivering even in the heat and humidity. When I went to use the latrine, situated in its own Quonset hut, the stench just about knocked my socks off. Inside were wooden box toilets to sit on with catch buckets underneath the holes. Flies and other insects swarmed around, droning and buzzing like something out of a Hitchcock movie. My God, I thought, why exactly was it that I chose to come to this place? Jammed up in a tent, cold-water showers, toilets from hell. And I had passed over the possibility of a couple of pleasant years in the Public Health Service for this? What could I have been thinking?

Not that there was much time to feel sorry for myself. Or much reason either. The choppers came in right over our tents, that first day and pretty much every day after that, the whine of the engines and flap-flap-flap of the rotors bringing a rush of corpsmen, nurses, and doctors running toward the helipad and the triage unit next to it. Sometimes it was one or two choppers bringing in a couple of soldiers with injuries that might have happened a half hour ago or maybe even just a few minutes ago. Sometimes more choppers landed and we'd have twelve or fourteen wounded troopers lined up on gurneys.

The first week I felt overwhelmed; I had never done anything remotely like this. But people helped, they showed me how to manage. I pretty quickly began to get efficient at it. You grab a patient, establish an airway, stop the bleeding, get an IV started. You decide the X-rays you need and what kind of specialist you might want. You make a quick analysis and plan your surgery.

From my journal:

September 16, 1966

Young boy—happened to be a Negro—shot in the right hip with God knows what. Completely shattered the femur close to the pelvis. It apparently exploded in him sending filth and gunpowder and mud all through his thigh, his lower abdominal wall, scrotum, and penis. Black filth. Sciatic nerve was blown out, as was his artery and two thirds of the skin of his thigh. Is this the right way to stop world communism? Feel like I should write a letter to Lyndon Johnson. Send him some pictures. Not adequate, of course, but at least that would be something.

There was the medical part of it. But then there was the human part. What could you say to these troopers lying there in front of you maimed. "Doc, I know they blew off my legs, but what about my balls?" What could you say? A soldier came in with a huge wound in his back. A rocket had hit him; the area around the wound was swollen grotesquely. He was going into shock, scared as hell. I jumped in and got an IV started. Boom, boom, boom. I was getting fast at this. He asked, "Am I going to make it, doc?" The universal question.

"Oh, yeah, you're going to be fine." I'm working this, that, and the other. "I'm going to fix you up, get you to the OR."

But he didn't make it. We controlled the bleeding. But it was too late; the physical shock killed him.

That night and the next day I thought about him, him and others I was losing, having this internal conversation with myself. You can do all this stuff. You're doing it well. You're good at it. But for some of them you're going to be the last human being they will ever see or ever talk to. You've got to say more than "You're going to be okay" and slam an IV needle in. You've got to take some time, you've got to look them in the eye and interact. You have to talk to this fellow human being who's lying there in shock and fright.

Sometimes there was the slack to do that. As far as the wounded went, it tended to be either feast or famine. Out there in the jungle beyond the city, the battlefield had its own rhythm. If there was a lull in the fighting we might be mainly taking care of people who were stabilized already and who were waiting to be airlifted to the U.S. hospital facility in the Philippines. Other times one or two helicopters would be coming in every hour or so. Then we'd all be working fifty or sixty hours straight, only snatching a brief couple minutes of sleep here or there. The rest of the time we were up to our elbows in blood. In those terrible periods I'd sometimes get to feeling as if my hands were operating on automatic pilot. I might be standing there semicomatose, my eyes glazing over, but my hands knew the debriding routine by themselves. Cutting, washing, clamping off arteries and veins, cauterizing bleeders.

Finding a way to deal with all this emotionally was crucial. If you allowed yourself to get dragged into thinking too much, you'd simply be crushed to pieces. I mulled over the idea of sending a letter and photos to Lyndon Johnson. I composed the letter in my head a dozen times, thinking about what words might have the most dramatic effect. I tried to figure out how I might actually get it to him so that he would read it. I imagined getting him and other world leaders down into a MASH unit operating room before they'd be allowed to start their wars. Grab them by the collar and force them to watch a terrified young man writhing in pain with his legs mangled or his belly ripped up. But of course that was just escapist fantasy.

The reality was that there wasn't the slightest thing I could do to stop what was going on.

But it went beyond that. After a while I began to think about the war from a political point of view too. Was it really worth all this carnage and death? Not just on our side, but on theirs, the Vietcong and the North Vietnamese? The fact was that I was treating their wounded right along with ours, in a guarded Quonset hut that served as the hospital's POW ward. All our docs were assigned there in the same way we were assigned to our own wounded, and we tended to their injuries the same way we tended to those of our own soldiers. With the language differences there was very little talking involved, but one injured VC I took care of had been a high school teacher and his English was pretty fluent. He wasn't even really Vietcong, he told me. He had just gotten completely fed up with Americans occupying his country, he said—and with the traitors who were running it, Thieu and Ky. "You are the aggressors," he said. "I'm not communist. I don't care anything about communism. I just want to liberate my country." His anger had welled up to such an extent that he left teaching and went off into the jungle. In his first firefight he had gotten half his ass blown away by a burst from an M-16.

What he said got me to thinking: How many other Vietcong were motivated the same way? And what did that say about our presence here? I had been going back and forth about the war in my head, but my talk with him was a tripping point, a trigger that helped me make up my mind.

Oddly, maybe, all this didn't fill me with a sense of futility. It didn't make me depressed or drive me into a state of frustration or rage. On the contrary, after a while it gave me a way to deal. I can't help these things, I began to think. I'm not going to be stopping the war. I'm not going to keep anybody from being shot. So, given those givens, let me do what I can, and that's it. Don't look at the things you can't fix. Look at the things you can. Just do what you can do and keep moving. Do today's work today, as the great Osler said. Don't think about yesterday, don't worry about tomorrow. Just do today's work today.

That mind-set gave me some peace. It made me think of another Osler quote, from an essay I had read in medical school that
had impressed me so much I even memorized a few lines. The essay
was called "Aequanimitas"—equanimity or imperturbability, which
Osler believed was the single most important quality a physician
could have. "No quality takes rank with imperturbability," he had
written. "Imperturbability means coolness of mind under all circumstances, calmness amid storm. Imperturbability has the nature
of a divine gift." How true that was. Calmness amid storm. What
could you need more in a place like Vietnam?

At some point pretty early on, I reached a kind of protective
equilibrium. It was possible to sympathize with these young men,
one after another shot all to hell. But too much sympathy meant too
much pain, which could make you nonfunctional in a matter of
days. It would turn you into a basket case. A little sympathy you
could allow yourself. More than that and you weren't doing anybody
any good. Not yourself, and certainly not your patients.

There was another element in the emotional equation too,
something that's a little hard to admit because it seems callous and
self-serving. I don't know if other doctors, especially combat doctors, have written about this, but it was part of my psychology about
what I was doing, and I'm sure it was for other docs too. That other
part was the nurses.

Those nurses were exceptional human beings. Most of them
were not career military but civilian volunteers, and almost all of
them were young. We doctors were in the operating room all day and
frequently all night too, doing surgery after surgery on young men
whose injuries would make your head spin if you didn't somehow
get yourself inured to it. I think that one way we did inure ourselves
was that we leaned on the nurses to provide the emotional care and
consolation that we couldn't. They were on the wards, taking care of
the soldiers. And they were good, not that they had any special training to do this emotional heavy lifting. But we knew the nurses were
going to look after them well, which relieved us of an emotional burden that would have been too much for us. And that burden truly

was on them (though I don't think many of them considered it a burden; compassion was a strong part of their makeup). We could slough it off onto them, but there was no one for them to pass it on to. The nurses were where the buck stopped. No one talked about this, but it was always there. It was a part of the psychological dynamic that enabled the hospital to run.

The nurses were magnificent. To me they were the true heroes of Vietnam, they and the helicopter pilots who brought the wounded in. Of course, I worked with the nurses and saw them all the time. I knew a lot about the pilots too, but I only had one firsthand experience of their bravery and skill—the time I went on my one and only medical foray into the field.

One afternoon word came that an orthopedist was needed to volunteer for a rescue mission. A trooper had fallen and broken his femur on a mountainside miles outside of Qui Nhon in a nonsecure area. They needed an orthopedist to splint the leg properly, then help figure out how best to get the trooper down from there.

I didn't even really think about whether I should go or not, I just grabbed some splints and jumped into the back of the waiting ambulance. We drove fast over the road that led west out of town, then onto rough terrain, rattling and shaking so hard I had to hold on tight to keep from getting tossed around. When we finally got to the mountain I knew there was no way the ambulance was going to make it up—the incline was much too steep. The driver did manage to get us up a hundred or so yards, then I hustled out, grabbed my gear, and ran off toward a trooper who was going to show me the way. Up above us on the little trail three others waited at intervals to guide me to their injured buddy, as if I were a baton they were passing along on a relay.

When I finally scrambled up to where the injured soldier lay, my breath was coming in whoops and I could hardly stand. But after taking a minute or two to recover I got to work, and with the help of a medic got a big Thomas immobilizing splint on the leg. Then we called in a medevac chopper.

We had the patient splinted and strapped onto a stretcher when the helicopter arrived. It hovered while the pilot looked for a place to put down. But there wasn't any. The mountainside was all rock and heavy bush, and far too steep for a landing. Slowly and carefully the pilot inched the chopper lower until the open hatch was about eight feet above the slope. There he hovered, almost dead still in the air, waiting for us to lift the stretcher up to the corpsmen in the hatchway. The long rotors were whipping around no more than two or two and a half feet from the side of the mountain. I would have been staring at them in horror except that the medic and I were too busy straining to hoist the stretcher up into the medevac corpsmen's waiting hands. I knew enough to know that if the chopper shifted and a blade hit the mountainside, that would be it. The chopper would have ripped itself up in a fiery crash, and us along with it.

Fortunately, there was no enemy fire. But I heard many stories from wounded troopers about pilots putting down in hot fire zones to take them out. This one relatively tame exercise was plenty for me, but the pilots did what they did day in and day out. They had courage I didn't know people were capable of. I don't know who showed more guts, the nurses, in their own way, or those pilots. In my book those were the heroes. In the middle of all that carnage they lit the place up with the power of the human spirit, what I began to think of as the human spirit indomitable.

As time went on I realized that I was seeing more wounded black soldiers than I might have expected. Blacks were 11 percent of the American population. I wasn't keeping count or anything, but I knew that a lot more than 11 percent of the wounded were black, which meant that a lot more of the dead were too. And what I heard from the black troopers was that they were more likely than not to be chosen as point men when they went out on patrol. It was easy enough to rationalize the numbers—lower socioeconomic groups tended to be better represented in the army and were drafted at higher rates. But in the operating room I wasn't thinking like a sociologist, I was just seeing what I was seeing. And what I was seeing told me that race meant something here. The army had been integrated for twenty years, but integration didn't mean that everyone believed everyone else was equal. And it wasn't just what I was hearing from black troopers. I was getting some of it myself too.

The Qui Nhon Officers' Club was one of the few local places that offered a chance for some decent rest and relaxation. Situated near the beach, it had a good view of the ocean. You could get a steak and a beer in there and even a bottle of champagne if you wanted. They brought bands in on occasion, so if you had a date you might even do a little dancing. Not that you often saw anybody with a date. American women weren't that common, so if someone did have a date it attracted a lot of attention.

That was a problem, especially for me. I did bring dates there a couple of times, but all my available dating partners were white— which meant we drew lots of extra attention. Some of the guys in there were just out of combat and were pretty gruff. They were also armed, all with their .45s on their hips, and they were drinking. One evening there was some unpleasant grumbling from a couple of officers who had just come in from the field. While I was dancing I heard, "You know what we'd do in the South. We'd just take him outside and cut it off," not loud, but loud enough for me to hear. My date was scared. Right then I thought prudence was the better part of valor, and I took her and myself out of there.

My problems along these lines came to a head when a delegation went to formally complain to John Feagin, an orthopedic surgeon who was our hospital CEO. They were upset that I was dating who I was dating and wanted John to put a stop to it. But they had misjudged their man.

John and I shared an office in one of the Quonset huts that also served as the workshop and storage area for casts. John had arrived in Qui Nhon shortly after I did and we quickly became good friends. Coincidentally, we were at exactly the same stage in our professional careers—we had both just finished our residencies. But John was career military; he was a West Point grad who had served three years in the artillery before the army gave him permission to attend medical school. As commanding officer of the 85th, he was strongly inclined toward academic medicine and he gave the facility something of a teaching hospital atmosphere. Doctors' groups made rounds whenever we were able, and John and I, at least, wrote several papers together that were published, one in the *Journal of Military Medicine,* another in the *Journal of Clinical Orthopedics.* Since we both had our orthopedic boards coming up, we did a lot of studying together.

John was a first-rate surgeon and an excellent administrator. Among his other qualities, he seemed to be completely color-blind. He was a white guy from Texas, but he had zero tolerance for what he considered racial bullshit. He told me that two factors went into his feelings about race. Here's how he explained it years later when I asked him specifically.

"One [this is John speaking] was that my dad was a career West Point graduate military officer. And one of the sharpest memories I have of him was the morning he left our house after strapping on his pistol. He was commanding officer at Hamilton Air Field at the time, in Marin, California. I had never seen him put on his pistol before when he went to work, and I never did after that day either. On his way out he said, 'Truman integrated the armed forces. I intend to see that this air base does it peacefully.' When he came back twenty-four hours later he said, 'It's done. No fights, no casualties.' He was expecting problems. He was amazed that nothing had transpired.

"That affected me deeply. So I always knew that the armed forces were integrated, and I believed in that. It was a matter of pride for me that my dad had taken a firm stand on that way back when. The second thing was that I was an artillery officer before I went to medical school. All that time I depended on black sergeants and soldiers and fellow officers. So that was my background on the subject."[2]

The delegation that knocked on John's door that night didn't know this about him. If they had, I don't think they would have shown themselves. They certainly wouldn't have told him that they wanted him to do something about me dating white nurses, "*our* white nurses," as they put it.

John was so inflamed by these people that he started looking for something heavy that he could do some damage with. He wasn't going to debate this or even listen to it. He was ready to shoot it out at the OK Corral. He told me later that he didn't feel like he was defending me so much as defending who we were as a hospital team dedicated to treating American soldiers, by which he understood *all* American soldiers, equally. That this kind of racial prejudice had reared its head in his command made him see red. And that it was happening in a combat zone made it a whole lot worse.

I tried not to get too worked up about these things myself. I was a free man. I was going to date whomever I wanted—even though prudence might steer me away from the officers' club. Not that I was happy about that, but I managed to swallow it. It didn't make much sense to go looking for a fight, especially not when people were drinking and armed. But there were some things I most definitely was not going to take.

A short time after I arrived, the doctors' living quarters got upgraded from tents to an officers' barracks a mile or so from the hospital. Most everybody walked to and from work, but I had a rare and precious commodity at my disposal—a jeep. I had the jeep due to a certain army organizational concept called the KB-Team. An orthopedic KB-Team consisted of an orthopedic surgeon, an anesthesiologist, a general physician, a couple of medics, some specialized equipment, a truck, and a jeep. For some reason—probably because I was fully trained—I was assigned as head of a KB-Team attached to the 85th Evac Hospital. Which is why I had the jeep, and why I drove to the hospital every day.

One morning as I was driving into the hospital area I saw a large Confederate flag adorning one of the outer Quonset huts. I wasn't in a happy mood to begin with, thinking about the war and the fighting and heading in to another day of wading in blood, and the sight of that flag just set me off. Mornings were always bad for me, and that particular morning wasn't any different. Damn, I thought. I've got to come in here and look at that thing? I jammed on the brakes and hopped out, ready for a fight. Maybe looking for a fight. I went into the hut without the slightest idea who I might find, maybe some colonel, maybe some angry redneck sergeant, I didn't care. In retrospect, I think this was bringing out all the anger and emotion I had been doing my best to keep tamped down.

Inside the hut a spec was sitting behind a desk.

"Hey, buddy, whose flag is that outside?"

"Don't know, sir, think it belongs to the sergeant."

"Where is he?"

"Over there, sir," pointing.

I walked toward the back.

"Say, sergeant, whose flag is that outside?"

"It belongs to the motor pool."

"Well, let me tell you, I didn't come over here to this God-forsaken place to fight for that flag. That's not my flag. I came over here to fight for the American flag! I don't know what that thing means to you. To me it means slavery. I'd appreciate it if you would take that thing down, right now would be a real good time to do it. I don't want to see that thing when I come back!"

I didn't stick around to watch. But when I drove home it was gone.

These kinds of incidents—the Officers' Club, the Confederate flag (there was another Confederate flag too that I asked to be taken down)—were upsetting; they had the potential to explode. But they didn't, and they were isolated episodes. A more general problem that I faced was the sense of disregard I picked up from some of my white fellow surgeons. I'm not talking about outright bigotry; in the operating room there was nothing so overt as that. But I was an anomaly at the 85th Evac Hospital. I think, in fact, that I might have been the only black surgeon in Vietnam. Stereotypes are tough to break free of, and the black stereotype in most of my fellow docs' heads didn't have room for someone like me. The result was that I sometimes found myself having to fight hard for my diagnoses and procedures.

From my journal:

August 27, 1966

So many white docs have never had to deal vis-à-vis a black surgeon who may question, challenge, or even criticize. There's been a recognition of black competence on the stage and on the athletic field, but not yet a respect for the possession of mental ability. It's an adjustment for some of them to have to deal with me on an equal basis. Must remain strong and willing to stick my neck out if I think I'm right. If this upsets white docs, I guess that's just the way it is. It probably shocks and perturbs many of them that I don't go overboard to be friendly, or that I don't soften how I present my medical opinions. Some are obviously prejudiced and downright resentful.

One soldier was brought in with what turned out to be a dislocated spine, which wasn't apparent immediately, since there was no obvious wound in his back. But something blunt had hit him a violent blow. The X-rays showed that one of the joints between two vertebrae had been knocked out of place.

The neck region of the spine is called the cervical spine, which includes the seven vertebrae starting at the base of the skull. After looking at the pictures, there wasn't any doubt, in my mind anyway, about what had happened. We were dealing with a unilateral facet dislocation in the cervical spine. The facets are thumbnail-size structures on each side of the vertebra that overlap the facets on the vertebrae above and below like shingles on a roof. They constitute the joints of the spinal column, linking the vertebrae together and allowing for flexibility.

The facets are kept in place by ligaments that hold the joint together. Something had hit this trooper hard enough to bang one of the facets out of place. Ligaments had been torn. Other ligaments had stretched tight, locking the dislocated facet in place. This was an extremely painful injury. The question was how to treat it.

One option was to operate, open up his spine and burr enough off the undislocated lower facet to allow the dislocated facet to settle back into place, then fuse it with a bone graft and wire it together. Major surgery. The other option was skull traction followed by a cervical collar. We could attempt to apply enough pulling force on the spinal column to make the facet snap back on its own. While the other surgeons were debating, I came to the conclusion quickly that we should try traction. I was sure of it. Wayne Southwick was one of the great cervical spine specialists. I had trained under him for three years and I had seen him perform this procedure. I hadn't done one myself, but I felt a lot of confidence in my judgment of how to handle it.

We had already shot the trooper with enough morphine to make him feel more comfortable. We had also put him in minimal traction to relieve the pressure and stabilize him. To do this we had placed tongs in his skull, then attached the tongs to a rope and pulley system with about fifteen pounds of weight at the end.

Placing tongs in someone's skull might sound horrifying to a layperson, but it's not unusual or all that difficult. The tongs themselves are like scissors reversed, so that the two prongs push toward each other. After you deaden the locations where you are going to insert them, you sink the anchors on both sides, cranking them down so they penetrate the scalp and the outer table of the skull down to about seven or eight millimeters. Then you lock them in.

Our soldier had the tongs emplaced. The critical decision now was how much weight to put on the pulleys. My memory, or my understanding, was that the textbooks recommended thirty-five to forty pounds, but we didn't have the books available, so we had no immediate way of checking that. In addition, this soldier was big boned and heavily muscled. I was positive it was going to take more than the textbook recommendation to pull the spine enough so that the facet would snap back.

As we got started there was a palpable air of skepticism around the operating table. No one there, not the general surgeons, not the neurosurgeon, not John, not the anesthesiologist had any experience with this procedure. And the consequences of using poor judgment could be considerable. Apply too much force and you could rip the tongs out of the patient's head. You could stretch the nerves, or the spinal cord itself. If that happened the patient could end up with neurological damage, maybe even partial paralysis. Too much force could dislocate the other side of the affected vertebra as well and damage the ligaments and tissues more than they already were. But I was confident that if we went slowly and carefully this would work. I'd increase the weights incrementally; I'd monitor each step with X-rays before adding more weight.

I'm not sure what the others thought. They had to deal with their reluctance about a procedure they weren't familiar with, that might have seemed radical to them. Then they had to deal with whatever unspoken doubts they might have had about me. The result was that there was a good deal of tension as we applied what we believed were the recommended weights. As I expected, nothing happened.

Then I upped it, ten pounds at a time. Nothing. We put on fifty pounds, which is considerable weight. Taking pictures on our portable X-ray machine, I could see some alleviation, or reduction, in the dislocation. The facets were moving, though very little. I could see the soldier's neck straightening—another good sign—but again, not much. I put on more weight. At sixty pounds I gave the patient an intravenous bolus of Demerol and muscle relaxant. I put on ten more pounds. Suddenly there was a loud pop, as if someone had snapped his fingers—the sound of the dislocated facet snapping back into place. Everyone in the room heard it, and the X-ray confirmed that the spine had regained its proper alignment. Gloating wasn't my style, but if it had been, that is for sure what I would have been doing.

That night I wrote in my journal about how appreciative I was of Wayne Southwick. The surgical training was one thing, but it was the attitude he instilled that I was really thinking about. He had allowed me to take the reins as a resident—in the old Halsted tradition. He had built my confidence. I had internalized his lessons about the necessity of thinking independently, of having the courage of your convictions and acting on them. That was the true hallmark of his mentoring. That was his standard, and the procedure that day made me feel I was learning to live up to it.

Many entries in my journal are brief:

October 8, 1966
Lots of traumatic orthopedics today.

March 19, 1967

Appreciate the rest from debriding gunshot holes.

May 14, 1967

This day was the bottom. Perhaps sickness, but more psychological. Fatigue and anxiety.

When I wrote in my journal that I was having a bad day, I meant it was a *bad* day. That meant that whatever was going on was depressing me, making me sorry I was there. Making me think, How many days do I have left to get out of here? I'm so tired of this blood and gore. I'm so tired of all this suffering. Other days were better. Doing good surgical work was satisfying. I saw exceptional examples of courage and strength every day, which lifted my spirits. But there was one aspect of my life in Vietnam that gave me a different perspective altogether.

When I first arrived in Qui Nhon, John Feagin's predecessor was still in command. This was Tony Ballard, a hand surgeon. "You know," he told me, "there's a leper colony nearby. It's not a secure area, but I've been out there a number of times. There's a lot that can be done. You may want to go out and see what's going on. Maybe you can be helpful."

I thought about it. How leprosy is contracted is not well understood. Prolonged intimate exposure magnifies vulnerability, but the vectors of contagion aren't clear. At the same time, sulfa drugs retard the bacteria's progress, and I was told that all the patients there were on sulfa. I thought it through and decided the risk was minimal. Besides, all doctors have a little bit of a missionary attitude. There's only an occasional Albert Schweitzer, but I think everyone would like to do at least something along those lines. "Yes," I told Ballard, "I'd like to go out there." So that's what I started doing.

The leprosarium was located on the beach eight miles or so from the city. It was run by nuns from the order of St. Francis, and the contrast between the colony and everything around it was stark. It was as different from the stressful and often depressing atmosphere of the hospital as you could get. Driving through the broken-down, shabby, war-torn, filthy village next to it, you would think you were in Soweto. But at the gates of the leprosarium another world opened up.

The first time I went out there I was amazed. The gatekeeper, one of the patients, took off his tattered brown felt hat and said, "Chau dong, bac si"—Good morning, doctor. Limping on damaged feet, he swung the gate open onto what looked like a movie set. The leper colony was beautiful, pristine. I drove up an immaculately kept sandy road, arched by palm trees; it actually reminded me of Stanford's Palm Drive. Beautiful little pastel-colored dwellings lined the street, all made of marble. The Qui Nhon region was a center of marble and granite production—which I hadn't known—and the patients supported themselves as marble workers.

There was a serene air about the place. The nuns who ran the leprosarium were an upbeat group. The patients, despite the severity of their disabilities and disfigurements, seemed cheerful and at peace with themselves. The thought struck me that something utterly different was going on out here, something almost spiritual. It was also obvious that this was a place where a surgeon could do a lot of good.

Before long I had established an informal routine. Subject to the workload at the hospital, I started going out to the leprosarium two half days a week. Since I was in command of a KB-Team, I could load up a truck with instruments and supplies, grab a couple of corpsmen, and get out there, sometimes with an anesthesiologist and another surgeon, sometimes even with a nurse or two. Everyone who went there felt good about it; they wanted to be there. When John Feagin took over at the hospital, he himself started coming out whenever his schedule allowed.

Because the leprosarium was in a nonsecure zone I was a little nervous about the Vietcong, especially when there was a flare-up of fighting in the area. I'd talk to the nuns and they would say, "It's okay. We're praying for you," which wasn't that much of a comfort. But we also knew that many of the patients had relatives who were Vietcong. That was our real security. We were helping family mem-

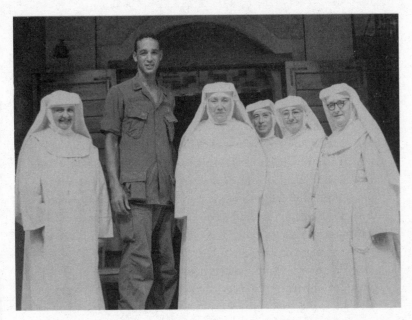

With Mother Superior (third from left) and a group of nuns at the St.
Francis Leprosarium (or Leper Colony), Qui Hoa, Vietnam, 1966–1967.
From the AA White Family Collection.

bers who were suffering from one of nature's most infamous and
mystical diseases. Despite my nervousness, I didn't really think anybody was going to touch us. And nobody did. None of the medical
people who went out there was ever harmed.

The major problem with leprosy is that it attacks the nerves,
including the sensory nerves. The bacillus infiltrates the ulna nerve
and the median nerve in the arm, and people lose sensation in their
hands. Imbalances in nerve function cause a "clawed hand" deformity. If fingers or a hand are injured, leprosy sufferers don't feel it.
They can use their hands as tools and it doesn't hurt. The damage is
cumulative, and over time they can lose fingers or even an entire hand.

In the feet it's the peroneal nerve that most commonly is involved. The peroneal branches off the sciatic nerve and supplies

movement and sensation to the lower leg, foot, and toes. When the nerve is damaged it causes what's called a foot drop. The foot drops down and turns in. With that condition, people walk on the sides of their feet, which damages them. They can step on anything sharp or abrasive and they won't know it.

The organism doesn't attack just the nerves, it attacks the blood vessels. It also infiltrates the skin, and even the bone to some degree. It cuts off the blood supply. When the blood supply stops, the area hardens up and eventually just falls away. Cheeks, noses, and ears lose their integrity. You see the awful leonine faces of leprosy.

When John Feagin and I first went there we were more interested in working on hands. Hands are more challenging than feet, more interesting surgically. There are procedures called tendon transfers, where you can take a claw hand and, by rerouting the tendons, you can significantly improve function.

But when lots of patients showed up with foot problems, we quickly realized that they felt it was much more important to be mobile. So we ended up doing almost no hand surgery but a lot of foot surgery, improving walking ability with a variety of procedures and educating patients about how to walk, to take shorter steps (which decreases wear and tear), and to protect feet and examine them for damage so that if an infection started it could be treated quickly.

I would bump along on the drive out to the leprosarium thinking about how at the hospital I was seeing the worst that man can do to man, then I go down the road and see the worst that nature can do. Man's inhumanity to man and nature's cruelty to man—both of them an absolute bitch.

Although triple sulfa drugs can slow leprosy down and may even temporarily arrest it, the disease is inevitably progressive. But it moves slowly. It gives its victims plenty of time to adjust to their circumstances. Just the opposite happens on the battlefield, where robust young men can find their lives devastated in the blink of an eye. Maybe that accounted in part for the tranquility and gentle demeanor of the leprosarium patients, their quiet determination. Here was yet another lesson for me in the human spirit indomitable.

I didn't know who was helped most at that leper colony—the helpers or the helpees. I hope I made enough of a contribution so that they got more out of it than I did, but I'm not sure of that at all. For me the St. Francis Leprosarium was an oasis; after all the blood and gore, it seemed almost a place of meditation. I came into a peaceful setting where all I had to do was what I knew how to do. I had everything I needed, and then some. Do you want this, *bac si*? Do you need that? Once I went into one of the operating rooms and bumped my head on the doorway. The next time I was there they had raised the doorway three feet, high enough for a giant to walk through. I had the pleasure of getting to know the nuns and seeing how happy they were in their vocation. I had what I can only describe as the joy of treating the patients, the most grateful patients a doctor could possibly have. In many cultures leprosy is regarded with such horror that if anybody just makes eye contact and looks at lepers and acknowledges them as human beings, they are profoundly grateful. And if you help them? You fix them up? You take care of them and look after them? The feedback is incomparable. The leprosarium refreshed my spirit. It helped keep me whole.[3]

I worked at the leprosarium throughout my tour. The day I went to say good-bye, the nuns invited me to have tea. Afterward I walked over to the ward to see a few of the patients for the last time. But as I approached the building, people started appearing from what seemed out of nowhere. Some limped or hobbled along on crutches. Some walked steadily, their feet improved by the surgeries we had done. Many had friends or family with them. It dawned on me that nearly every patient I had treated in the course of my visits was there. They had elected a spokesman, John Noel, a half-French, half-Vietnamese former pharmacist. He began, but he was obviously nervous and emotional, and his English faltered. He just couldn't get out what he wanted. "*Bac si*, number one, *bac si* number one," he said. But that wasn't enough. Finally he just pointed at me. "You," he said. "You Muhammad Ali." That was about the best I have ever felt in my life.

Shortly before my tour was up I received an enthusiastic letter from Wayne Southwick, telling me that the NIH grant to study biomechanics in Sweden seemed to be firming up. I had been thinking about what should come next, and the idea of going into private practice was getting to seem more attractive than it previously had. Given everything I had gone through in Vietnam, I wasn't sure I was looking forward to another year of training. But when I discussed it with John Feagin, he said, "Are you crazy? You mean you have a chance to go to Sweden to do a research fellowship and then go back to Yale, and you're actually thinking about it? You must be out of your mind! Of course that's what you should do!" It was with that piece of advice ringing in my ears that on August 7, 1967, I flew out of Saigon's Ton Son Nhut airport bound for Tacoma, Washington, where I intended to kiss the ground the moment I got down from the plane.

6

GETTING TOWARD EQUAL: SWEDEN

We started at the top of the medical profession millennia ago.
Though we have not been there since, we have been contributing
all along and are on our way.

—W. Montague Cobb

AT THE END of my tour, I wrote in my journal:

August 6, 1967
Said I'd give Uncle Sam a good hard year's work, and I did. Grateful
to be alive—and whole.

I was so grateful, in fact, and so happy and relieved to be back, that
when the plane landed at McChord Air Force Base in Tacoma I did
get down on my knees and kiss the ground.

I had actually been back to the States briefly a number of
months earlier when I tended a badly wounded soldier on a medical
evacuation flight to Walter Reed Hospital in Washington, D.C. I was
in Washington for two days then, enough time to meet with Lent
Johnson, a prominent orthopedic pathologist at the Armed Forces
Institute of Pathology whom John Feagin said I should look up. I
also wanted to meet Montague Cobb if I could. Montague Cobb had
been in the back of my mind ever since Walter Greulich, my old
anatomy professor at Stanford, had mentioned him. "Make a note of
it," Professor Greulich had told me. "Dr. Cobb is a close friend of
mine. It will be good for you to get to know him."

Montague Cobb, MD, PhD, was a professor of anatomy at
Howard University. Walter Greulich had thought he might be an

important person for me, since Cobb, an African American, was one of the world's leading anatomists and physical anthropologists, a true giant in his field. I was a freshman medical student when Greulich and I had had this discussion, a little lost, like many first-year students, and in need of encouragement. Greulich knew I wouldn't be encountering many black professors on my way to getting trained, and he thought that Cobb would be an inspiration for me. Unfortunately, I'd never gotten to Washington to meet him. Now seemed like a good opportunity.

Lent Johnson at the Institute of Pathology knew Cobb and gave me his home number. When I called and introduced myself, telling him that I'd been referred by my former professor Walter Greulich, Cobb said, "Of course we can meet. How about tomorrow at my club?" That was how, the next day, I found myself having lunch with Montague Cobb at Washington's famous Cosmos Club.

Cobb was then in his mid-sixties. A stocky, muscular-looking individual with glasses and a warm expression, he shook hands firmly and welcomed me to the club. Right from the first moment it was apparent that he was pleased to see me, which was especially gratifying, considering I was the one who was so pleased to meet him at long last. Yes, he and Walter Greulich had known each other for ages. Did I know how his old friend was doing? He was glad I had met Lent Johnson. But most of all he was glad to know that I was making my way as an orthopedist, that I seemed to be surviving well and moving along through the system. "We're getting a few people accepted into medical schools now," he said. "We've opened a hole in the line. What we need to do now is get as many people through the hole as possible, before it closes back up."

I knew Cobb's reputation as a scholar and teacher. At Howard he had assembled one of the world's great collections of human skeletons for the study of comparative anatomy; he had authored a prodigious number of papers, textbook chapters, and monographs; he had been instrumental in building up Howard's medical school; he had served as editor of the *Journal of the National Medical Association* for years and had written for its pages what amounted to a history of black American medicine. The man was, simply, a phenomenon.

He was also a racial pioneer, with a string of "firsts" behind him. But what I didn't know then was much about his activities as a civil rights fighter. I learned a great deal about that part of his life later on, but looking back, it's a little embarrassing to think how little I knew when we first met.

The fact was that Montague Cobb was the embodiment of the scientist as social activist. In addition to his numerous research papers on general anatomical and clinical matters, Cobb authored medical-anthropological studies about the myths of black/white mental and physical differences. But his chief focus as an activist was racial discrimination in health care. He saw the ghettoization of black medicine as the major culprit in the inferior state of health among African Americans. Black patients and doctors in American hospitals suffered from pervasive discrimination. Righting that injustice was Montague Cobb's personal crusade.

Through the 1950s many hospitals either were segregated completely or had special segregated wards for black patients, and not just in the South. The major federal hospital legislation, the Hill-Burton Act of 1946, actually endorsed the "separate but equal" policies that were, of course, separate but not by any stretch of the imagination equal. Black doctors found it next to impossible to get staff positions or privileges at hospitals, which often meant they couldn't get their patients admitted or even referred. Black physicians were excluded from the American Medical Association and many of the other professional societies. Only a few mainstream medical schools had any black students at all and, as I knew so well myself, the number of black faculty members was next to nil. In effect, the health-care system simply did not recognize the idea of equality for either African American patients or doctors.

To help counter all this, in 1957 Montague Cobb launched a major assault on hospital segregation. He called it the Imhotep National Conference on Hospital Integration. Imhotep was the father of Egyptian medicine, which the ancients considered the world's most highly developed. And the ancient Egyptians, whatever their actual racial identity might have been, were definitely people of color, "dark of skin," as Cobb put it. "Therefore," he said, "we claim him."[1]

The Imhotep conferences were held from 1957 through 1963. The NAACP sponsored them, along with the Medico-Chirugical Society of the District of Columbia (the country's first black medical society) and the National Medical Association—the African American counterpart to the whites-only AMA. The mission of the conferences was to bring together all the organizations, interest groups, and government agencies that figured into the problem of hospital discrimination; to define the problem, publicize it, and find solutions to it.

The first Imhotep Conference invited all the organizations that composed the American medical establishment. Not a single one sent an accredited representative. But Cobb was relentless. He lobbied for legislation, he brought legal actions, he gave speeches, he published articles and pamphlets. He held more conferences. He didn't stop until the Civil Rights Act of 1964 made segregation in hospitals illegal. Actually, he didn't stop then either, because although hospital discrimination against black patients and doctors became illegal, it did not just suddenly disappear.

Sitting across from Cobb at the Cosmos Club, I thought of him as an inspiration, but mostly in personal terms. He was a famous medical scientist and a renowned professor, a black man whose life shone with accomplishment. But I didn't grasp then that the man I was having lunch with was a key figure in the great post–World War II civil rights revolution. He hadn't received the national publicity some of the civil rights leaders had, which was why his contributions weren't widely known. But they were essential. In 1947 Truman had integrated the armed forces. In 1954 Thurgood Marshall brought the *Brown v. Board of Education* case to a successful conclusion, and school segregation was outlawed. And all that while

Montague Cobb was fighting for equality in another major dimension of American life—health care.

Cobb was a leading lobbyist for the 1964 Civil Rights Act that put an end to so much of the de jure inequities that limited the lives and aspirations of African Americans. I can't say that I was thinking about these things in any kind of comprehensive way back then. In 1966 I was a twenty-nine-year-old combat surgeon. I mainly had two things on my mind—Vietnam and my upcoming orthopedic board certification exams. But whether I or any other particular individual was looking at the big picture wasn't the point.

The point was that even with the postwar advances, racial prejudice was something that reached into everyone's life, white and black. For people who grew up when I did, thinking in racial terms was inescapable. It was in the air everyone breathed. If you were black you thought about it in one way, if you were white you thought about it in another. But black or white, you thought about it. It was part of your psychology, always there, in the front of your mind if you lived in a place where the races mixed, in the back of your mind if you were from Nebraska and never met a black person. It inhibited personal interactions and distorted professional relationships. Racial prejudice was so ingrained that it seemed normal. Sometimes it was subtle, sometimes not. Either way, it tainted the atmosphere.

I had learned to cope pretty well, I thought. But I understood the deep psychological hold of racism only after I had the chance to experience life in a place where skin color wasn't right up front on everyone's radar screen. Actually, it had never occurred to me that there might really be such a place, although I had heard a certain amount of talk about how liberal Sweden was. In any event, the subject wasn't on my mind as I prepared to leave for the University of Gothenburg where, thanks in large part to Wayne Southwick's advocacy, NIH had come through with a fellowship for me at Carl Hirsch's biomechanics laboratory.

Shortly before I left for Gothenburg I received a telegram from Professor Hirsch's office advising me to get in touch with a

Sister Kerstin at Carlanderska Hospital who would arrange living quarters for me. I was shocked to see this. "Appalled" is probably a better word. "Sister Kerstin," the telegram said. The last thing in the world I expected was to be living in some kind of convent attached to what I supposed must be a Catholic hospital. I had visions of myself in a sparse, cell-like room, living among the sisters of whatever order they had over there in Sweden. I mean, I had gotten along wonderfully with the nuns at the leper colony, but Sweden was supposed to be a free and easy place. I was looking forward to having a social life there, which wasn't very likely if I was going to be living in a convent.

When I got to Gothenburg, though, I found to my vast relief that Sister Kerstin wasn't a nun, Carlanderska wasn't a Catholic hospital, and my living quarters weren't in a convent. It seemed that in Sweden all nurses were customarily referred to as "sister." Sister Kerstin was the chief nurse at Carlanderska, in charge of housing among other things. My apartment, a spacious flat on the beautiful, manicured hospital campus, was ordinarily set aside for the physician-in-residence. By American standards it was more than adequate. By Swedish standards, as I came to understand, it was luxurious.

Carl Hirsch, when I met him the next day, did not look at all Swedish, or at least not what I thought Swedes were supposed to look like. He was short and dark, with heavy brows, deep-set eyes, and a long face. He spoke quickly in a resonant voice, welcoming me in perfect English. It wasn't just his English that was perfect. I had heard that he lectured worldwide in German, French, Spanish, and Norwegian, in addition to Swedish and English. He spoke Yiddish too, and apparently gave speeches in that language when he visited Israel, though not to scientific audiences. Sitting there, I was more than a little in awe; Hirsch was the world guru of orthopedic biomechanics. But I felt comfortable too. There was a twinkle of warmth and enthusiasm in his eyes. Great men in European universities were supposed to be haughty and aloof. I didn't know if that was true. But that was pretty obviously not Professor Hirsch's style.

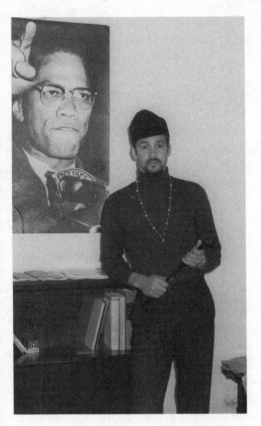

In my apartment at Carlanderska Hospital, Göteborg, Sweden, 1969. From the AA White Family Collection.

There was something else I picked up from that meeting and my subsequent meeting with Hirsch, when he showed me the laboratory and we talked over the research I might be doing. I thought back to my first meeting with Wayne Southwick and to my other residency interviews. At Yale, race was an issue. When I had sat down to interview at Mayo, at Columbia Presbyterian, at Harvard, and at all the others, I felt it, as did my interviewers, all of them distinguished department heads. Though it was hardly mentioned, race was the 900-pound gorilla sitting there with us. With Carl Hirsch there was nothing. There was his professional interest in me as his new American researcher, his personal interest in making me comfortable as a visitor in his country, and nothing else. The race gorilla wasn't there. Hirsch didn't notice, he didn't care. He wasn't the slightest bit interested.

And it wasn't just Hirsch. Something different was going on in this place. I could tell that to some people I seemed a little exotic. Negroes were a rarity in Sweden, and the Swedes weren't color-blind. But that was it. Black, white, no one seemed to care one way or another. I don't think they would have cared if I was purple with green polka dots. I was just . . . another person.

You have no idea what that meant. It was like being free of some curse, not having to scope out the setting on the color meter everybody you met was sure to be carrying around with them. As I got to know my colleagues in Hirsch's lab, people at the hospital, neighbors, no one was overeffusive, no one was confused or muddled, no one was skeptical or antagonistic. No one was anything but normally friendly. They were pleased to meet me. That was it.

That was an amazing, liberating feeling. And nowhere was it more amazing than when I met women I wanted to ask out. Once when I was on a brief R-and-R leave from Vietnam I had met an American girl from the South. This was in Hong Kong. We had hit it off almost instantly. We liked each other, we spent the day together sightseeing and having fun. Then in the evening over dinner she told me I looked Puerto Rican. Was I Puerto Rican? "No," I said. "I'm black." "Oh," she said, slumping down in her chair and starting to cry. "Are you absolutely sure?" And that was that. But in Sweden, women couldn't care less. It took some getting used to.

But it wasn't just women. Nobody cared. When people said hello, it was just hello. Not hello—I see by the color of your skin that you are a white person; what kind of white baggage might you be carrying toward me? Or, hello—I see by the color of yours that you're black; wonder what kind of baggage you might be carrying toward *me?* We'd better be a little careful until we can sort this out.

As I was absorbing all this, I was also taken by another element in Swedish culture that had me thinking. At the medical center where I was working, every morning I passed by a dignified middle-aged gentleman wearing a suit and bow tie, which seemed to be his trademark. Each day we greeted each other politely as we passed by, a friendly "good morning." I hadn't met him formally, and I assumed he must be one of the administrators or perhaps a doctor or scientist. But one day I noticed him wearing a janitor's blue jump suit, emptying a trash bin. He wasn't an administrator or a scientist, he was a custodian. Each day he came to work, took his suit off in the locker room, put on his janitor's uniform, and did his job.

I realized that what had struck me was the way he carried himself with such dignity and self-esteem. Without his uniform he was indistinguishable from anyone else at the center. As I got to know Sweden better I realized there was nothing unusual about this. The country had an egalitarian feel about it. People didn't try to put themselves ahead of others. They tended to accept each other as equals in a way I wasn't used to. Drawing attention to your accomplishments, or even your children's accomplishments, wasn't the norm. The norm was to see yourself as just a regular person. When the son of one of my colleagues scored a hat trick at a soccer game I watched, the congratulations were more reserved than they would have been at home. He had done something exceptional, but that didn't mean he should be elevated too high above his friends and teammates.

From what I could see, Swedes didn't have a compulsion to make themselves out as better than someone else. For an African American who grew up in segregated Tennessee, that was dramatic. In Memphis, black subservience was expected. Race made all the difference, and class made a difference, and class and race reinforced each other. But in Sweden there wasn't even the vast differences in wealth, at least not that I could see. I knew there must be very rich people here, but most everyone seemed to live more or less the same way. I thought, I'm in a country where egalitarian values are lived, not just talked about.

As I absorbed Sweden's egalitarian ways and Swedish people's coolness about race, I also started reading. For the first time in my adult life I had the leisure to explore subjects other than medicine. Maybe it was too late for me to become an intellectual, but at least I could start filling in some of the gaps.

I wanted to understand more about politics and economics and about how societies worked. I considered myself a humanist, a black humanist, but what did that mean? Humanism was a way of relating to others. But that had to be based on a deeper understanding of others than you could get just through personal experience. I was stimulated to read not just by my own curiosity but by the African students in Gothenburg I was getting to know. I was impressed by how much more knowledgeable they were than I was, or than the guys I knew at home, white and black. It was as if while we had been talking about sports and music, their routine conversations had been about politics and racism. In our discussions they would roll out historical facts about Europe and Africa, about colonialism and liberation. They were used to talking about these things. They were far more globally aware than we were.

So I began reading about communism and capitalism. I picked up books on the black experience: Eldridge Cleaver's *Soul on Ice*, Price Cobbs's *Black Rage*, Frantz Fanon's *The Wretched of the Earth*, Gunnar Myrdal's *An American Dilemma*. Then out of the blue I had my first up close encounter with the violent edge of the American struggle, in the person of Bobby Seale, cofounder with Huey Newton of the Black Panther Party.

Sweden, when I arrived there, was a country angry about the Vietnam War and consequently highly critical of the United States. Sweden gave refuge to American military deserters and provided assistance for North Vietnam. One result was that American antiestablishment figures came to visit and give speeches and interviews, which were widely covered. One of these invitees was Bobby Seale.

Of course, I knew about the Panthers. I admired Seale and Huey Newton for their guts in standing up to the establishment. I had never met anybody associated with them, but I had become friendly with a few ex-pat brothers, including Solomon Pelham, who had been in the air force. Solomon was surviving on the margins in

Sweden, but he was very bright and one of the world's great conversationalists, and Solomon had some connection to whatever group it was that had invited Bobby Seale to Gothenburg. The group couldn't have been well funded, because although they had invited Seale, they weren't able to get him a hotel room, which Solomon told me. And since I had room, I told Solomon that Seale was welcome to stay with me. That's how Bobby Seale became my roommate for a week.

Seale had some speeches and media interviews lined up, but he had a lot of down time too, and we spent much of it talking. Seale was obviously bright and courageous. Although he was a leading militant and I was nothing of the kind, he never spoke down to me or tried to show off or exalt himself. On the contrary, he listened to my experiences and thoughts with respect. I sensed that he was a decent person, but a decent person caught between a rock and a hard place.

What I heard from him was that the Panthers' protection was beginning to run out. They had been the darlings of the American Left, but the violent defense of black people they advocated and some of the actions they undertook were undermining their support. Seale felt the party was under siege. He thought it was time to pull in their claws and become less aggressive, a course he wanted to follow. But the way you moved up and demonstrated leadership in the Panthers was by being as radical and militant as you could. So Seale was faced with a group of younger, even harder brothers trying to push him out. He was struggling to navigate that, and the pressure was telling on him. He talked about it and drank while he was talking. He ran through various fifths of Scotch during the week he was there with me, trying to wrestle with his problems.

Seale wasn't the only militant I got to meet. Miriam Makeba, the famous South African singer and one of my all-time favorites, came to Gothenburg to give a concert. She was married to Stokely Carmichael at the time, and he was there with her. One night I found myself in a room with Solomon Pelham and two or three others listening to Stokely expound.

I don't know if Stokely Carmichael was the first black activist to use the slogan "Black Power," but that's what I associated him with. I knew that he had marched with Martin Luther King and that he had done a lot to register black voters in the South. I credited him for that. His was a bold voice. But whatever his accomplishments might have been, that night his talk sounded out-and-out crazy. He told us his plan was to get into Togoland and take control there. Once he had done that, he was going to use Togoland as a base to organize the continent and develop a pan-African revolution.

I asked him, "Stokely, where are you going to get the guns and all the other things you'll need to do that?" I didn't know about revolutions; maybe he did have resources. But he couldn't answer my question. That was his vision. That was his plan, and that was what he was going to do. It sounded completely off the wall.

"Yeah," he said at one point, "these young brothers come up to me and say, 'I want to be part of the movement,' I tell them, 'Look, I don't know who you are. You go out and ice a pig, and then you can come back and talk to me.'" He was serious. I thought he might be borderline insane. Looking back at the militant black leaders from those days, I would guess that he was not one with the strongest IQ, or the strongest mental hygiene either.

Personally, I had seen more than enough violence to last me a lifetime. I didn't need any more of it. I wasn't impressed by what I was reading about communism either. From what I could see, it had at least one fundamental flaw. I didn't enter much into the heated political discussions going on around me, but my own conviction was that communism was doomed. I thought it denied the individual's striving, competitive human nature, the desire to lead, to stand out, to satisfy the need for personal fulfillment.

Egalitarianism was one thing. I loved the way that was built into Swedish culture. I wished we had a lot more of it in ours. But in Sweden, egalitarianism appeared to coexist nicely with meritocracy. Nowhere was that more evident than in the Swedish medical science community, at least in orthopedics. Getting to know some of my closest colleagues in Gothenburg and later at the Karolinska Institute was a humbling experience. I am not exaggerating when I say I sometimes felt almost overwhelmed with gratitude that I had found my way there. I couldn't believe that I had almost passed up the opportunity.

It wasn't only Carl Hirsch, the world leader in his field. Another close colleague and friend was Alf Nachemson, whom I met only a few days after I arrived in Gothenburg. Alf was Hirsch's star protégé. Hirsch had noticed his exceptional talent while Alf was a medical student. Not someone who believed in wasting time, Hirsch had arranged for Alf to graduate early so he could get on with the business of making an impact on the world of spine research and treatment, which he quickly proceeded to do. His PhD thesis on measuring pressure inside the lumbar disks was an experimental breakthrough in managing back pain and provided standards that are still operative a half century after his initial work.

Then there was Bertil Stener. If Carl Hirsch didn't look Swedish at all, Bertil Stener looked like an advertisement for Swedish manhood. He was six three, erect of stature, broad of shoulder, and blond of hair. He had high cheekbones and what my mother used to call "carved features." I wandered into his office one day looking for a tennis match. Somebody had told me that he played. I myself had played for years every chance I got. After I was done with my college athletic career I still felt the need for some hard physical activity, and tennis filled the bill. I may not have been a great tennis player, but I thought I was pretty good. I wanted some competition.

With Bertil I got more competition than I bargained for. He was a good deal older than I—thirteen years to be exact, but he was a step faster, he hit a little harder, and he never, ever put the ball anyplace other than the absolutely most effective place. Damn, he was good. Unbeatable. At least I never beat him. And if anybody else ever did I'd like to hear about it. "Gee, it was funny to play with you," he'd invariably say after winning yet another match. By which he didn't mean that my efforts amused him, but that playing with me had been a lot of fun, a sentiment so innocent and genuine that my feelings about losing to such an older person would vanish in the air.

With Bertil Stener I felt an almost instantaneous sense of collegiality and rapport. Something just clicked, from our first tennis game until his death thirty-plus years later. I came to think of him as a true soul brother. He had various large talents that complemented his skill at tennis. But it was his mastery of orthopedics that made him famous.

Bertil was a phenomenally gifted surgeon. Among the procedures he practiced with such consummate deftness and grace was the single most difficult operation known to man: the total spondylectomy—that is, the intact removal of malignant tumors of the spinal column by removing the entire bony structure of the spine where the tumor is located, including removing it from around the spinal cord itself.

Bertil pioneered this procedure, developed it, and taught it. He devised ways of protecting the spinal cord while removing the bony structure. He excised the diseased region, then reconstructed the spinal column to his own design, masterfully carving bone grafts or donor bone and inserting them together with plates, wire, and screws to reconnect the two ends of the severed spinal column. Nature then did its healing work, so that in time the patient would be able to walk and live a near-normal life instead of dying from the malignancy.

These operations took thirty to forty hours. Bertil spent weeks planning all the details. He happened to be a superb artist and would draw the diseased spine with the tumor, draw the excision he was planning, then draw exactly where the transplanted bone, wire, plates, and screws were to be placed for the reconstruction. Spine surgeons throughout the world viewed his work with awe. At one presentation he made to the Scoliosis Research Society using slides, X-ray pictures, and personalized clinical reports and photographs of patients who had survived fifteen years or more, he received a thunderous standing ovation. I have never seen nor have I ever heard of anything like a standing ovation for a clinical presentation.

Wayne Southwick's idea for my Swedish sojourn was that I would spend some time with Carl Hirsch, familiarize myself with orthopedic biomechanics, and take a look at how biomechanics might relate to clinical practice. Then I'd come back to Yale, beef up our teaching in that area, and see if we couldn't get a biomechanics laboratory started.

But Hirsch had a different view of what I should be doing. "You ought to do a research project," he said, "something that will result in a doctoral thesis."

I wasn't planning that, but once he mentioned it I thought that maybe this was an opportunity to investigate some fundamental orthopedic questions I'd had in my mind. What's the most important thing in orthopedics? I asked myself. Maybe bone healing—fracture healing. A big unanswered question in this area was whether bones heal better by intermittent loading or by rigid immobilization. That is, is it more effective to treat a fracture by putting a cast on it or by using a plate or rod to rigidly fix the bone in place? A cast allows for intermittent pressure: think of someone walking with a leg cast. A plate or rod immobilizes the fractured bone. We were treating them both ways, and no definitive, comparative, experimental studies had been done. They've got this really great lab here, I thought. I could do animal studies and figure it out. That would be a significant contribution.

That was my idea. But Hirsch thought I should expand my thinking. Yes, bone healing was important. On the other hand, he was enthusiastic about work that some of his PhD students had done on spinal kinematics—detailed analyses of how the spine's joints move under normal circumstances. That was fundamental knowledge the profession needed to have. Once we fully understood movement, we would be able to make far more cogent judgments about treatment options. "We've developed the technology for these studies," he told me. "And we've determined the detailed, three-dimensional kinematics of the cervical spine. We've done a lot of work on the lumbar spine too. But you know, Gus, nobody's yet looked at the thoracic spine, and, of course, that's where most scoliosis exists. So, we have the technology. We can get the specimens. The work's just waiting for someone to do it."

Well, that was interesting. They had studied movement in the cervical spine (the upper seven vertebrae) and the lumbar spine (the lower five vertebrae). But normal movement in the thoracic spine—the middle twelve vertebrae—that was uncharted territory. And after three or four meetings with Hirsch it dawned on me that maybe he didn't actually want me to do a fracture study, and I suddenly had an aha experience. Aha, I thought, what I really ought to be doing is a kinematic study of the thoracic spine. That could be incredibly fruitful. Why hadn't I thought of it earlier?

With that settled, I learned the technique, rolled up my sleeves, and went at it. Hirsch and one of his students had developed an experimental apparatus that allowed for precise measurement of spinal motion. The spine specimens themselves came from fresh cadavers. Spinal segments were excised in the autopsy rooms of local hospitals, sealed in plastic, and frozen. When I was ready, I unfroze them and prepared them for our experiments in a specially constructed high-humidity chamber. We had learned that keeping the segments moist was key to maintaining their original flexibility.

After I prepared the segments I set them up on our apparatus, which allowed me to make precise measurements of movement in both two dimensions and three, using X-ray pictures, displacement gauges, extensometers, and other measuring devices. The various measurements were recorded electronically; then I put them through a mathematical analysis on the big mainframe computer we had access to.

In the end, I believed, I would be able to present a clear, precise, and comprehensive picture of the normal movements of the thoracic spine. Doing that would enable clinicians to better understand the diseases and traumas they treated clinically; it would give them a baseline. You have to be able to understand the normal before you can understand the abnormal. As one researcher wrote, looking at the disease process without reference to normal function is like trying to understand an accident simply by studying the wreckage.[2]

This was exciting stuff. The information I was generating would help orthopedists to make better judgments about treatments. It would open avenues for innovations and discoveries. I did all the experiments, I collected the data. But some of the analysis resisted my efforts. I was dealing with sophisticated concepts of force and displacement, engineering concepts really. Okay, Gus, I thought, you've gone about as far as state-of-the-art orthopedic biomechanics is going to take you. Now you need an engineer.

It wasn't easy convincing Carl Hirsch of this, though. He had supervised dozens of PhD studies, all of them without getting any engineers involved. He knew more or less everything there was to know about biomechanics. The idea didn't particularly appeal to him. But I was persistent. "This is as far as we can go, professor," I told him. "We do need an engineer."

I'm not sure if I persuaded him or just wore him down, but finally he said, "Okay, why don't you go over to Chalmers and get one"—the Chalmers Institute, Sweden's MIT, was located nearby. So I did. After a couple of visits to Chalmers I came back with Manohar Panjabi, a doctoral student from India in mechanical engineering.

My new engineering partner and I moved the work forward. We were able to extract more useful data and more precise data from my numbers. I was able to put the presentation into a theoretical construct that fit engineering thinking. A year and a half after I arrived in Sweden I was ready to publish and defend my thesis.

With the publication of *Analysis of the Mechanics of the Thoracic Spine in Man*, I felt I had made a real contribution to orthopedic medicine. I had a new sense, too, for where I might be heading in my professional life. But as I got ready to go back to America, I found myself thinking that the most significant thing about my experience here wasn't the science I was able to do.

"To be completely candid," I wrote to my mother, "I have to say that the time I have spent here has been the happiest in my life. It has been an opportunity to see a different set of mores at work, to see ideals in action. Most of what I learned here has to do with a philosophy of life. I have a lot more of an idea of where I am philosophically, politically. I have a clearer idea of the goals I seek. It has strengthened my resolve to do things." Along with the letter I sent

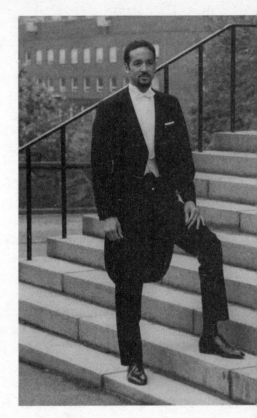

In characteristic Swedish academic disputation attire, Stockholm, Sweden, 1969. Photo by Bertil Stener.

her a copy of the thesis. It was dedicated "To my mother, my late father, and to all Afro-Americans."

In December 1969 I defended my thesis in the time-honored Swedish manner. Dressed in white tie and tails I stood at the podium in an auditorium at Stockholm's Karolinska Institute. Carl Hirsch had moved from Gothenburg to Karolinska, so that was the venue for my defense. On either side of me sat a professor, similarly attired. They were my "opponents," formally charged with disputing my methodology, my analysis, my conclusions, and my presentation. It was a ritual that went back to medieval times. My thesis itself had been nailed to the door of the auditorium for the past two weeks for public examination, just as Martin Luther's theses had been in Wittenberg in 1517. In the audience sat Wayne Southwick, who had flown over from New Haven. I think he was impressed by the proceedings, which were a good deal less pompous and severe than the formality suggested. Swedes always like to inject some humor into even the most serious events. "You look good, Gus," Southwick told me afterward, admiring my outfit. "Maybe we should institute the same kind of thing at Yale."

7

A MAN AIN'T NOTHIN' BUT A MAN

I have adjusted my thinking . . .

—Malcolm X, on his return from his pilgrimage to Mecca

I HAD WRITTEN TO MY MOM from Sweden that my year and a half in that country had given me a better idea of where I stood politically and philosophically, that I was clearer about what my goals were. One of those goals was to do what I could toward diversifying the Yale medical school student body, by which I was thinking specifically about getting some more African American students in there. That one-black-student-every-other-year business still rankled. I didn't think that particular unwritten understanding was still in effect, even though there were still only a few black faces among the med students, which told me that nothing much had really changed, despite the ten or eleven years that had passed since I had first interviewed.

With that in mind I gave a call to Jerry Burrows, a friend who had been chief resident in medicine when I was chief resident in orthopedics. Jerry was now chairman of the admissions committee. "Of course," he said, when I asked if I could join. "Happy to have you."

So, diversity was now formally on my personal agenda, at least diversity as I was thinking about it at that point. But Wayne Southwick had not brought me back to Yale to advocate for diversity; he had brought me back to move the department ahead in orthopedic biomechanics, to teach it and to set up a lab, if I could.

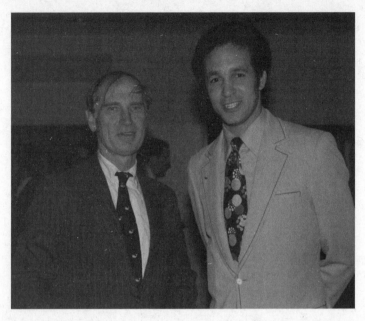

With my mentor, Professor Wayne O. Southwick, Old Lyme, Connecticut, 1978. From the AA White Family Collection.

To our knowledge, there were only one or two significant biomechanics laboratories in the country, including the one Victor Frankel and Al Bernstein ran at the Hospital for Joint Diseases in New York, where Wayne and I and our other colleagues had taken that course before I went off to Vietnam.

In terms of getting our own lab started, there were only two problems: money and space, neither of which the orthopedics department had available. Wayne wanted it, I wanted it; we thought the medical school needed it. But without money, the idea was a nonstarter. We needed a grant. I started writing proposals, but what with my new teaching and supervising duties and my operating schedule, the time I had for this was limited. Additionally, many of the NIH requests required preliminary data, which I, of course, didn't have yet. So the lab idea seemed to be at an impasse, until divine intervention appeared in the persons of Alfred and Blair Sadler, universally known at the medical school as the Sadler twins.

The Sadler twins were Yale Medical School administrators who ran the Physicians Assistants Program, a two-year training program to qualify bright young people to work as doctors' assistants, teaching them how to take histories, do physical exams, order lab studies, and in general extend the reach of physicians, both primary care and specialist. The program incorporated lots of clinical experience and turned out graduates who were almost on the level of doctors, except without the medical science knowledge. The Sadlers had asked if I could help with admissions screening and some teaching for this program, and I had volunteered.

Somewhere in the course of working together I had told the Sadlers about our hopes for an orthopedic biomechanics lab, and also, I'm sure, about our impoverished circumstances. And they said, "You know, we actually have some money you could use. Not much—only ten thousand or so—but we could definitely arrange it."

"Oh, thank you very much," I said. "That's great." On the one hand I was grateful for their offer; on the other, I wondered how far ten thousand dollars was going to get me.

Then I thought of Manohar Panjabi, my engineering partner back in Sweden. Before I left I had had dinner with him and his wife, and he had said in passing something about how he would like to go to the States one day. Ten thousand dollars was a pittance. But Manohar had just finished his doctorate. He was probably still living on his Swedish student's stipend, which couldn't have been much. Manohar was a first-rate scientist; his English was excellent; he had truly enjoyed the biomechanics work we did; he was attracted to the United States. Maybe ten thousand would be sufficient to bring him over long enough to get things started.

At the end of the academic year I made time to visit him in Sweden. "All I have is ten thousand dollars," I told him. "But if you come over, our job will be to work like hell and try to get some grants. If we succeed, we can support you with the grant money. You could think of it as a one-year fellowship. I wish I could offer you more, but if we're successful, it will be a different story."

"Well," said Manohar, "I think I could do that. Why not?"

I couldn't have been happier. Given that Manohar had a wife and two children to support, his willingness to take a leap into the blue like this showed a lot of courage and confidence, which stoked up my own optimism. Having Manohar along gave me a real shot in the arm. With him on board, I was sure we'd have a good chance of doing something truly important.

That summer I had a special visitor from Sweden, Anita Ottemo. Anita and I had met while I was working for Carl Hirsch. We had liked each other tremendously and had been dating for four or five months before I had to get back. The first time we met, we were having coffee together, and when she smiled at me I thought, Okay, this is definitely the girl I am going to marry. A cliché feeling if there ever was one, but the fact was I did have the strongest conviction at that moment that she was the one. Of course, I hadn't told her that. But apparently the attraction was mutual, and now that I was established in New Haven we were seriously considering getting married. But first Anita thought she had better check out the country. I had loved Sweden. Whether she might love the United States was an open question.

Once I knew Manohar was coming, I took Wayne Southwick up on the small junk-filled room he had managed to find somewhere in the upper reaches of Silliman Hall. When he first showed it to me, I couldn't even look because it was so depressing. Maybe twenty by fifteen, the room was filthy, full of dust and grubby, old, broken-down equipment. But if Manohar was going to come, we needed something, anything, so this room would have to do.

I poked in there with Anita while I was showing her around and said something about getting the janitorial staff up here to clean, that once we did that it would probably make a decent little laboratory. The next thing I knew, Anita took the room in hand herself. Anyone who knows something about Scandinavians and cleanliness

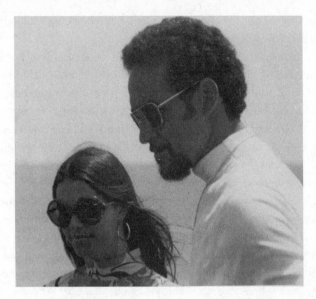

With Anita Ann-Katrin Ottemo at Newport Jazz Festival, 1970. Courtesy of Charles McWhorter.

will understand that when I say the room was pristine when she was done, what I mean is that you could eat off the floor. I wouldn't have thought twice about performing an operation in there.

Anita's efforts didn't only unclutter the room, they uncluttered my mind. Suddenly I could see how we really could set a lab up in that space, and I began to get excited about the kinds of experiments we might do, especially once Manohar was on the scene. I even started on a couple of minor studies before he arrived, helped out by a technician who gave me some time and by several student volunteers. Then, when Manohar did arrive, we started working like mad on grant applications. We were also able to collaborate with the neurosurgery department on a project that the chief there, Bill Collins, had succeeded in getting a substantial grant for. Then we received our own NIH multiyear grant to explore fracture healing—my old interest. With that, Manohar and I were in business. We started to build what would eventually become a leading center for the study of orthopedic biomechanics.

Four years later Manohar and I used the expertise we had accumulated to start writing a text on the biomechanics of the spine. That was a prodigious undertaking. Quite a lot of papers and monographs had been written on the subject, a substantial number by Carl Hirsch and his many students, but no one had ever undertaken to survey the whole field and present the available knowledge in usable, textbook form. Given the scope of the project, I might have been a little more cautious. But Don Nagle, a Yale professor when I was a resident, liked a particular saying that was almost like a mantra for him, that he'd repeat often to his students: "Make no small plans. Reach for high ideals and high goals." I thought that was pretty good advice, and I had internalized it. The textbook idea fit right in. In the end, it took Manohar and me two years and more to complete the book, but it did become an essential text. We dedicated it to our families, and to Mahatma Gandhi and Martin Luther King.

RIGHT FROM THE START I loved being on the Yale faculty. I enjoyed the collegial atmosphere and felt at home there among the university's libraries and laboratories. I got great satisfaction from my research, and after a year-and-a-half break in Sweden I was especially happy to be back to the operating room.

Teaching also gave me real gratification. Mom and Addie had been teachers and I'm sure some of their love for it had rubbed off on me. I also admired the great teachers I myself had been exposed to, and I had always tried to understand the characteristics that made them so effective. In addition to my classroom teaching, I inevitably found myself mentoring, or at least interacting closely with, the school's few black students. From time to time I'd have lunch with them in the cafeteria, where they had a habit of clustering together and segregating themselves. I thought that was fine, but I'd also tell them how extremely important it was for them to get together with their white classmates. "You want to make a contribution, you want to do something for your race in the future? You should welcome the opportunity for friendship and mutual respect with your other classmates. The chances of one of us ending up as secretary of health, education, and welfare is pretty slim compared to the chances that one of your other classmates will. So it's a no-brainer. Don't isolate yourselves. Nothing wrong with hanging out together, but make the effort, reach out." I said that a lot. It *was* a no-brainer.

I also invited the great Montague Cobb to Yale for a lecture. Secretly, in my own mind, I brought him there to inspire the black students, and also to show him off in front of the white faculty, many of whom, of course, did not know about him.

Yale might have been a cathedral of learning, but it was no ivory tower, most especially not in 1970. That year—this was shortly after I got back—New Haven was practically exploding, and Yale was exploding along with it. In May four student war protestors at Kent State were shot dead by National Guard troops, an event that galvanized the already volatile antiwar movement, including in New Haven. On top of that, the city was the scene of another galvanizing event, the Black Panther murder trials.

Interestingly, New Haven was famous for another court case that had pitted black defendants against the government. A hundred and thirty years earlier the *Amistad* trial had been held there. That was the case where a Spanish slave ship bound for Cuba had been commandeered by its cargo of captured Africans, who killed the captain and forced the crew to sail them back to what they thought would be Africa, but which turned out to be the United States, where the vessel was seized by a U.S. warship off Long Island Sound. The Africans were accused of murder and piracy by Spain, which demanded their extradition. The American government wanted to comply, but was stopped by a court case brought by abolitionists, who eventually won the Africans' release.

The Black Panther case was far different but may have been at least equally emotional, if not more. Seven Panthers were accused in the killing of another Panther member whom they believed was an FBI informant. Two other Panthers were also tried, my former companion and temporary roommate, Bobby Seale, and a young woman named Erika Huggins. Seale had given a speech at Yale the day of the murder, and one of the arrested Panthers had said that he, Seale, had personally given the order to kill the alleged informant. The same arrested Panther accused Huggins of helping to torture the dead man prior to his murder.

The arrests and trials in this case caused an eruption of rage on the part of students and others sick and tired of the war and completely fed up with the Nixon administration and J. Edgar Hoover's FBI, which had gathered some of the evidence. Thousands of protestors poured into the city. Major antiwar figures, including Benjamin Spock, Abbie Hoffman, and Jerry Rubin, addressed the crowds. Kingman Brewster, Yale's president, announced that he was skeptical that black revolutionaries could get a fair trial. Yale's nationally known chaplain, William Sloane Coffin, said, "All of us conspired to bring on this tragedy by law enforcement agencies by their illegal acts against the Panthers, and the rest of us by our immoral silence in front of these acts." The students went on strike, the police used tear gas, bombs were thrown at a local skating rink.

So, there I was in the middle of all this uproar. I didn't condone violence, and most certainly not murder, but there was a general feeling that the trials were based on manufactured evidence, and two of the accused, Seale and Erika Huggins, hadn't even had their day in court yet; they were being held in pretrial detention, where they'd been for some time. My own emotions were right up there on the surface—all that personal history of needing to do something for the race, all the frustration of not having ever actually done much at all, my sensitivity to the activists' repeated charge that middle-class blacks like myself were "bougies," bourgeois sellouts who were comfortable with their own privileges and didn't give a damn. All that together with my admiration for the guts the Panthers showed in standing up to the establishment and pushing for black rights—which they were demanding right now, not later. So I thought, Okay, what can I do? I'm no gun-toting revolutionary, but how can I be supportive?

Back when I was an intern at Michigan, when Martin Luther King was starting his marches, Reuben Kahn had told me to get myself trained and established first, then I'd be in a position to do something that would make a difference. Well, as a new junior faculty member I wasn't exactly well established, and I didn't know if I could make a difference. But at least I could do something. And when word got out that Erika Huggins was in pain in her jail cell and wasn't getting adequate medical treatment, that was my chance.

The American Medical Association had a dictum at the time: "Every American has the right to choose his own doctor." I grabbed onto that, and I thought, Okay, that's an American right. Should a person be deprived of that right because she's in pretrial detention, while she's innocent in the eyes of the law? If you're innocent until proven guilty, then why should you be denied the right to get appropriate care from your own doctor? What if all the black doctors in New Haven got together to insist on Huggins's right to see a physician of her choosing? Number one, that would be doing something for her, and number two, it would be a symbolic, humanitarian, public act of support for the black struggle.

Mobilizing New Haven's black doctors wasn't difficult. There were only ten, and three of us were connected with Yale: myself; Jim Comer, a psychiatrist who was serving with me on the admissions committee; and Marshall Holley, who had trained there in obstetrics—and Marshall had grown up in New Haven, so he knew all the local practitioners.

We met at the home of Dr. Fred Smith, an elderly family doctor in Milford, just outside the city. He was well known in New Haven, not just as a longtime local physician, but because for years he had made himself available to people in jail who needed a doctor. The other five or six had various specialties, but everyone there was of one mind when it came to the issue at hand. They all felt almost exactly as I did.

Getting everyone on the same page was only a matter of connecting the dots. We were physicians. As physicians, here was something we could do that was in our field and would show our concern.

"This will be public," I said. "We should expect that we'll be involved in a legal battle. All of our names will appear in the newspaper at some point. In fact, we should make sure that they do. If anyone isn't comfortable with that he should say so."

No one said so. They all wanted to be counted.

I had already talked to Erika Huggins's attorney to get some guidance on how to go about this. Then we consulted with a local African American lawyer, who volunteered to handle our situation pro bono. We offered our services to Erika Huggins, who was glad to accept the offer. Then a couple of us arranged to have a friendly luncheon meeting with the state commissioner of corrections. This was a very polite, very proper meeting. "Sir," we said, "we are Ms. Huggins's doctors. We would like to examine her in prison and undertake whatever treatment might be necessary. She is in a good deal of pain and the prison health services are simply not satisfactory. We'd like to offer this as a humanitarian gesture."

The commissioner listened politely, and said No, just as politely.

"Please understand," we told him, "we will be pursuing this further."

Since we were preparing a test case, our next step was to go to the prison and be formally turned away. We went, and we were turned away.

At this point we contacted the newspapers with a letter all ten of us had signed. "Brothers and Sisters," we wrote. "We, the undersigned black physicians, because of our concern that you may not be given adequate health care, are offering you our services free of charge. We are aware of the inequities in health care in the black and other economically deprived communities in our largely inhumane society... We feel that there should be special concern for your health... We are at your service." The letter was published. News articles appeared about the State of Connecticut prohibiting Huggins from receiving adequate health care. Then we went to court, asking for an injunction forcing the prison authorities to permit us access to our patient. The court rejected our appeal, declaring that this was a federal matter and that we would have to pursue it in federal rather than state court.

In the end the federal court granted the injunction, and Dr. William Massie and I were allowed in to see Huggins. We examined her and found she had an arthritis problem that was affecting her knee. We prescribed anti-inflammatories, which we felt would alleviate the pain. She was grateful for the visit, and for our offer to follow up and see her again if she felt she needed us, either in prison or afterward. And that was that.

Medically, this was not a complicated situation. But we all felt good about what we had done. We had come together as a group and had made our point. We had stood up. I'm sure that each of us thought of this effort a little differently, at least in terms of whatever it might have meant in our individual experience of racism and our place in the struggle to improve conditions for our people. Looking back, I think it was important that I was able to express myself—at least to some extent—in public. It was the first time I had done that, and I thought it was about time I did.

MEANWHILE, I WAS ALSO taking a more active role in trying to inject more diversity into the Medical School. I had received a letter from an old Mt. Hermon friend who lived in Chicago, Dr. Don Chatman, about an intern at the Michael Reese Hospital there who he thought would be an excellent candidate for an orthopedic residency at Yale. The intern, Carlton West, had been a top student at Morehouse and president of his class at Meharry Medical School. Chatman wrote that West was a young man of outstanding personal qualities as well as someone who had great potential as a surgeon. Might there be a place for him at Yale?

When I spoke to Wayne Southwick about West, he said, yes, he'd be able to work him into the residency rotation. But residents' salaries, as I knew, were paid not by the Medical School but by Yale-New Haven Hospital, and there were no extra salary slots available. Wayne would have to talk with Charles Womer, the hospital CEO.

The background to this is that Yale–New Haven Hospital served what was even then a fairly substantial black population as part of its patient community. In fact, the hospital was located directly adjacent to New Haven's working-class black neighborhood. In recent years Yale–New Haven had undertaken a public relations campaign espousing its commitment to inclusivity, outreach, and diversity. But though I was on staff and in the hospital every day, I didn't see that there was much, if any, progress in that direction. I thought the rhetoric was pretty hollow.

When Wayne came back from his meeting with Womer, he told me the president had refused to fund a salary for West. To say I was frustrated by this would be a major understatement. Here they were, claiming they wanted more minority staff doctors and residents, yet doing nothing to achieve that. And now they had a concrete opportunity to bring in a first-rate black resident, and they were turning it down. I was sure they could dig up the money for this. A single resident's salary wasn't going to break anybody's budget. As far as I was concerned, this was just so much blatant hypocrisy.

I knew Wayne wanted West—there was nobody more on board regarding diversity than he was. But Wayne was the only one on the surgery faculty pushing this issue, and he had only so much political capital. I didn't get the impression that he was willing to go to the mat for this. So I asked if he would mind if I talked to Womer myself. He didn't, and two days later I was in Womer's office making my best attempt to stay polite, but at the same time express how upsetting and insupportable this decision was, and why. Surely, I said, given Yale–New Haven's sincere desire to increase its diversity, and given that here was an outstanding candidate, Dr. West, who had the full support of the orthopedic chief of service—surely the hospital would be able to find the minimal funds necessary to fill this slot.

I thought I was doing a fairly good job of keeping my voice under control while I was telling him this, but I was staring him in the eye, and it's possible my face might have betrayed something of what I was feeling. It was clear from his own expression that he wasn't in the least happy to be listening to this, one of Yale–New Haven's very few black physicians in effect accusing the hospital of deviousness and bad faith. When I was finished, I heard this reluctant grumble from him that he would think about it. Then he curtly told me that he was sure I had a busy schedule, as did he, so "thank you for coming in." I didn't try to extend the visit.

Strangely, maybe, as I left I had a certain amount of confidence in the outcome. Despite Womer's obvious reluctance, I didn't think he'd want any more pressure to start popping up around this. I was also absolutely sure that if he looked hard enough he'd be able to find that one meager salary. And sure enough, the next day Wayne heard that a slot for Dr. West would be available.

Carlton West did a magnificent job as a resident and went on to become a prominent orthopedic surgeon in Chicago and a highly regarded doctor to celebrities. The fact was that getting him admitted was relatively easy. Wayne supported it and the hospital had put itself on record about wanting to increase its diversity. That was an individual case, though. It was a lot harder making any impact on the institutional selection procedures.

My first experience with this was as a member of the medical school admissions committee. The admissions process at that time was that each member of the committee would be assigned a certain number of applications to examine and candidates to interview. Then the members would present their applicants to the whole committee for discussion, ranking them low, medium, or high.

This process turned out to be intriguing and unpredictable. Some committee members, for example, were partial to musicians, so they might advocate for an outstanding violinist. Another firmly believed that captains of undergraduate sports teams were especially qualified. Others might favor entrepreneurial types, or student council leaders, or research types, or straight 4.0 students. It was so interesting to see the various committee members evincing recognizable patterns of advocacy. And since most of the candidates had excellent grades, test scores, recommendations, and so on, the

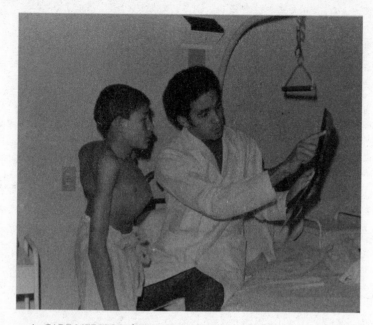

As CARE MEDICO Volunteer Consultant, examining a patient with a severe spinal deformity in Tunis, Tunisia, circa 1971. From the AA White Family Collection.

discussions had a tendency to turn lively and sometimes sharp. If we had admitted two football captains already, the musician advocates would be clamoring loudly for their candidates. I couldn't for the life of me figure out how we would accept Student A, a Phi Beta Kappa honors graduate in biology who had played violin for a year with the Philadelphia Symphony Orchestra but reject Student B, also a Phi Beta, et cetera, who had won prestigious prizes as a classical pianist. The answer seemed to be that after we admitted Student A, the sports enthusiasts would insist on the next football captain who was also Phi Beta Kappa, so Student B was out of luck.

Jim Comer, a young assistant professor of psychiatry, and I were the two African American members on the committee of twenty-five or so—actually, we were the only two African American medical school faculty members. Like everyone else, we were assigned applicants randomly. But we made it a point to become familiar with the black applicants, so that we could advocate for the especially good ones, which we did. There had certainly been no voice for them before, which was one of the reasons Jerry Burrows, the admissions chairman, had invited us on.

One aspect of some black students' applications that Jim and I noticed—at least applicants coming from the historically black colleges—was a quirk in their letters of recommendation. Many of these students were magnificent, wonderful academic achievers, athletes, musicians, what have you, but their letters of recommendation just seemed to be lacking in that extra firepower. The praise was there, but it seemed slightly grudging; it didn't match the effusiveness common for top students from other schools. This made it relatively difficult as Jim and I tried to present a case for these students as compared to others.

The two of us talked about this phenomenon, conjecturing why the faculty brothers and sisters at the historically black schools just couldn't seem to "give it up." My opinion was that it was a residue of what the great Caribbean psychiatrist Frantz Fanon, in his book *The Wretched of the Earth,* termed the "colonialized mentality." Fanon's point was that colonialized people, subordinated, oppressed, and defined as inferior, will begin to see themselves in exactly that light. They will themselves come to believe that their oppressors are indeed smarter, more talented, and more accomplished, while they are inferior and less capable. Then, as a psychological defense mechanism, they will identify with the oppressor, attempting to mimic and adopt the oppressors' behavior patterns, ideas, and attitudes, including looking down on their own compatriots. These psychological constructs, says Fanon, are deeply ingrained and largely unconscious.

Fanon was writing about Algerians and their French colonial masters, but I thought a great deal of his analysis was pertinent to our own situation here in America. That was why, I believed, our faculty references found it so hard to give full praise where praise was so obviously due. I'm happy to say that in the years since I was on that Yale committee we seem to have evolved a good deal farther away from Fanon's colonialized mentality paradigm, though we still see vestiges of it—sometimes significant vestiges.

The bottom line was that Jim Comer and I (with Jerry Burrows's cooperation) were able to substantially increase the number of African American students admitted to the medical school. We provided informed advocacy for a group that previously had not had anyone to speak for them. We were able to read between the lines of those recommendation letters and we were able to talk about the distance many of the African American students had traveled in their academic and personal lives, which often spoke to their determination and courage. Jerry Burrows, the chairman, supported us in good measure, though the attitudes of our other co-committee members could be mixed. The whole process illuminated for me how discrimination can and does happen, even where there is little overt prejudice at work.

When it comes to school admissions, employment opportunities, and other competitive situations, candidates from mainstream groups have natural, inevitable advocates, which minority groups simply do not have—unless institutions make a special effort to include them. It's an aspect of what writers like Allan Johnson and Tim Wise call "white privilege," or "white male privilege," the underlying advantages, most often unspoken, that differentiate dominant from subordinated groups.[1] I wasn't aware of these sociological analyses back then, but Jim Comer and I saw how it worked close up while we were on that admissions committee.

Sometime later I also joined the committee that selected interns and residents for the department of surgery. The selection process there echoed the problems of the medical school admissions committee, but it was a lot less civilized, and potentially more volatile. Also more humorous, in hindsight, anyway; though I don't recall being amused at the time.

There were seven of us on the intern and resident selection committee (I was the only African American), and each of us got to review essentially all the application dossiers. Once that was done, we brought all the dossier folders into the surgery conference room and put them down on a table in the center, arranged alphabetically. Then the fun began. Each committee member would pick up folders, look at the names, and put them in one of three piles: high, medium, or low. Committee members would be walking around the table picking up folders and prioritizing them, initially from the alphabetical pile in the middle, but then, when that gave out, from the high, medium, and low piles.

In the process, committee members would sometimes move dossier folders from one pile to another, indicating their disagreement with whoever had put a folder in a particular pile in the first place. Just as often people would move folders back to the piles they had originally put them in, indicating their disagreement with the disagree-ers. Not infrequently, I would be moving minority candidates up, but someone else might move them down, at which I'd move them up again. All this was happening with the seven of us circling the table in one direction or another, providing plenty of opportunity for people to get in each other's way or bump into each other. No words were exchanged—nobody talked at all while this was going on, but there was a lot of silent fuming as committee members watched each other reorder the choices they had made.

As the tension mounted I began to think that someone might physically attack me, and I got myself ready for it. Or maybe I'd even lose it myself and attack someone else. This is crazy, I thought, but then again, why would I be there and not do what I thought was right? No doubt others felt the same. Eventually, most of the members were more or less satisfied, or at least ready to compromise. The chairman resolved unresolved selections. Tempers cooled down. We took some good black candidates whom we certainly wouldn't have taken if I or somebody else of my persuasion hadn't been there. My memory is that the next year they changed the procedure, which cut down on the anger and frustration. But the playing field itself was nowhere near level until the institution made a formal decision to pursue diversity as an objective, and that was a good deal later on.

Yale was, and is, a progressive institution in many ways. But racial issues popped up, and I tended to be involved in them, or if not involved in them, I at least knew about them. In terms of my professional life, I couldn't have been happier, but that nagging racial dimension created a usually distant but always audible drumbeat. Sometimes I could barely hear it; other times, like when I was on those admissions committees, it was much louder. But the racial push and pull was usually institutional and almost never overt, which is why one particular incident seemed so bizarre.

By 1974, Manohar and I had moved the biomechanics lab from its original tiny quarters to the newly constructed research building. We now had a state-of-the-art facility, including offices for each of us and for our secretary/administrative assistant, Audrey Mendel, an efficient, hard-working woman in her late fifties who cared a great deal about the lab and about Manohar and me personally, her "children," as she thought of us (we thought of her as our Jewish "mom"). One day a junior faculty member who was running his own laboratory in the building, but with whom I rarely had any interaction, stopped by our offices for something. He was bright and energetic, but he had a kind of cocky, aggressive personality and what I thought of as a loose hold on propriety. When Audrey told him that neither Manohar nor I was in, he said, "Oh, who are they screwing now? That's probably all he"—nodding toward my office—"knows how to do. Screw." Then he laughed at what he must have considered a witticism (given orthopedists' use of screws, plates, and rods) and strolled out, leaving Audrey dumbstruck.

A day or two later she told me what had happened; I think she wanted to let her own emotions cool a bit. She was shocked that anyone would say something like that to her, and she was appalled by the racist nature of it.

I never had a quick temper, but this just flooded me with anger. I couldn't imagine anything like this happening. Who would ever say such a thing to me? And this was, if anything, worse. I mean, saying it to my secretary? I needed to impress on this individual that what he had done was outrageous, totally out of bounds. I was going to make that extremely clear to him. I thought, okay, no punches; I'm not going to hit him—unless he throws one at me. I'll try to avoid a fistfight, but God knows, if this guy starts something, he'll wish he hadn't.

I headed down toward his office, thinking that maybe I'd haul him out of his chair and read him the riot act. But as I got near his office, there he was, coming from the other direction. Perfect. He was already standing up. I wouldn't have to yank him to his feet.

I think he was a little surprised when I walked right up to his face, grabbed him by the collar with both hands, and jacked him up as high against the wall as I could. "Don't you ever!" I said. "Don't you ever talk to my secretary the way you did the other day! I can't believe you said that! You should be ashamed. I'm advising you never to try something like that again. Do you understand me? Ever!" Then I dropped him to his feet, turned around, and walked away. And that was more or less the last we had anything to do with each other. He certainly never came up to our offices again. This happened in the Yale University Medical School Department of Surgery in 1975, a place where I felt accepted, supported, and valued. But who knew what might have been going on under the surface?

TO PUT SOME PERSPECTIVE ON IT, while I was intensely aware that I was a *black* physician, what I tried my damndest to stay focused on was my life as a surgeon and professor. That meant constantly sharpening my skills, broadening my repertoire in the operating room, and working hard to be the best teacher and mentor I was capable of being. What helped immeasurably, of course, was that among my colleagues, present and past, were some true luminaries of the surgical world, people like Alf Nachemson, Bertil Stener, and Carl Hirsch (all of whom I eventually invited to the United States as visiting professors), and, of course, Wayne and my old teachers Victor Richards and Don King. So, I had plenty of models, and I

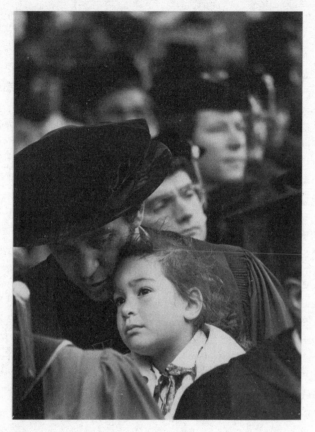

With my daughter, Atina (age six), during Brown University Commencement Ceremonies, June 1982. Atina later graduated from Brown in 1998.
Photo: John Foraste/Brown University.

did my best to live up to their expectations. I also had, in Wayne Southwick, the finest example of mentoring anyone could possibly have.

In 1975 my efforts along these lines paid off when I received an American Orthopedic Association ABC Traveling Fellowship along with three other young American and two Canadian orthopedic surgeons. These fellowships, awarded every two years, give upcoming North American surgeons the ability to travel to Great Britain to meet with, observe, and exchange ideas with leading orthopedists and orthopedic scientists there. I was intensely proud that I was the first African American surgeon to be selected for one of these prestigious fellowships. Our group went to London, Edinburgh, Bristol, Cambridge, and Oxford, among other places. The six-week trip was fascinating medically and socially. I think we all came away from it with important professional insights as well as an expanded sense of international collegiality. I also left England thinking about how rigid the class hierarchy still was there, and how relatively less difficult it was to break through social and economic barriers in the United States.

I think the visibility I got from the ABC fellowship and from some other circumstances contributed to a call I got from Brown University, my alma mater, inviting me to join the board of trustees for a four-year term. This was an honor I never anticipated and that I was hugely grateful for. At Yale I was moving up through the ranks, from assistant to associate professor, with an excellent chance, I thought, of making full professor, and maybe somewhere down the road even chairing a service or a department somewhere. But I didn't expect anything like a trusteeship, or the opportunity it gave me to really look into a university's inner workings—not to mention giving something back to my old school.

That was an eye-opener on many levels. The trustees got to talk with students, administrators, and faculty about how they saw the university and its procedures, its social dynamics, the effectiveness of its teaching—almost every significant dimension of what it meant to run a large, complex educational institution. And all of this, especially our meetings with students, including African American students, made me start thinking about diversity in a much broader way than I had been up till then.

At Yale I considered myself an advocate for diversity. By which I meant, specifically, bringing more black students into what was an almost completely lily-white environment. My main idea was to wake Yale up to the fact that there were excellent, deserving, qualified African Americans who, for a variety of reasons, were more or less invisible to the admission process. I wanted those young people to have a chance rather than no chance. So that's what I was aiming at.

But Brown was putting a different spin on diversity. Diversity wasn't at the top of Brown's list of concerns, but at least it was on the list. They had a campus committee on diversity issues; we, the trustees, had students come in to talk to us about it. Brown was definitely ahead of the curve.

The concept of diversity at Brown was beginning to evolve around one question in particular: What is the educational value of diversity? The idea was coalescing that diversity enriches the educational experience of everyone involved. There wasn't 100 percent agreement on this. Some of the students we talked with took a cynical view of the idea, a few black students in particular, who told us that they weren't there to educate white folks; they were there to accomplish what they wanted to accomplish. But that was a very small minority view. Many more students and faculty bought into the idea that all people in an educational setting should be willing to share knowledge with one another and learn from one another and teach one another, to achieve better understanding of cultural differences and the implications of them, and to appreciate the importance of working together and getting beyond the isolation of cultures from each other.

That concept was a lot different from just trying to get more black students accepted, which was where I was starting from. For the first time, I began looking at diversity as an inclusive social issue rather than mainly as a matter of achieving fairness for a dispossessed minority. Not that the two were mutually exclusive—far from it. But my instinct told me that viewing the question from the perspective of how diversity benefits the entire community provided a powerful and convincing argument for inclusion—of African Americans, but also of other minorities. Diversity was a black question, yes, but not only a black question.

My involvement at Brown drew me farther into this subject than I might have gone otherwise. But I was also reading a book that in a way bore on something similar. Reading isn't the right word; I was devouring this book. I was immersed in it and by it. I couldn't put it down. The book was *The Autobiography of Malcolm X,* written with Alex Haley.

I was, first of all, taken by Malcolm's incisive analysis of black America's white problem, his straightforwardness, his articulateness and courage in calling things out as they were. I felt emboldened by it. I wasn't about to go off and become some kind of crusader, but the book inspired me to at least act as forthrightly and assertively as I could in my own little sphere of influence.

Not least, I was fascinated by Malcolm's pilgrimage to Mecca and what had happened to him there. In Mecca he experienced the kindness and generosity and spiritual fervor of Muslims of every possible ethnic, racial, and national background. Mecca awakened him. It shocked him with the shock of what you could only call the brotherhood of man. Mecca ignited in Malcolm a transition from the black racial focus of Black Muslim Islam to the broader, nonracial, universal orientation of traditional Islam. And I thought, Wouldn't it have been nice if Bobby Seale had been able to retreat from his radical posture as gracefully as Malcolm was able to do through his pilgrimage. I saw that as Malcolm's epiphany, his revelation, his strategy, call it what you will, his opportunity to say that I can move from where I used to be to something larger and more powerful. It's time for me to do that.

I thought, You know, I've seen the same kind of thing. In a different way, of course, but basically the same. When I came out of that carnage in Vietnam, I came out with an even stronger sense that in the final analysis we are all so much more similar than different. Once you make the incision, once you look inside, everybody is the same. Open up that skin and underneath it's all one. The reality of the body tells this to you. It's a reality doctors see constantly. Our humanness supersedes our cultural issues, our difference in status or rank, our racial selves. A superior officer, a trooper, black, white—under the knife they're all the same, just as in pain they're the same. We all have our limits of pain, our levels of anxiety. Pain is an equalizer, and, of course, the greatest equalizer of all is death, of which I saw plenty. Death is *the* equal opportunity employer. In the final analysis that's all we are—human. A man, in John Henry's enduring words, ain't nothin' but a man.

For me, that was Malcolm's essential lesson. Being a trustee at Brown made me think about some of what that lesson meant in the university world that was by now my home ground and in the life I had chosen for myself as a physician. Although I didn't see it yet, it was a lesson that was going to shape a great deal of my own future.

8

ORTHOPEDIC CHIEF: HARVARD

Diversity should be a core value in the health professions.

—The Sullivan Report, "Missing Persons:
Minorities in the Health Professions"

THAT FUTURE BEGAN to reveal itself with a phone call I received one morning in the late spring of 1978. A Dr. William Silen was on the line. Dr. Silen introduced himself as the chief of surgery at Beth Israel Hospital in Boston. Of course, I knew of Beth Israel; I had a couple of friends who had been there, one on staff, one as a resident. Beth Israel was one of the major Harvard Medical School teaching hospitals. "I'm chairing our search committee," Dr. Silen said. "Beth Israel is planning to build a full academic program in orthopedics." The search committee wanted to interview me for the position of orthopedic surgeon-in-chief for the service. Might I be interested? This would be an important, ground-floor opportunity.

When I got off the phone with Dr. Silen, I just sat there for a moment, a little stunned. I loved Yale, where I had not too long before been promoted to full professor. But Silen was talking about a chair at Harvard, as chief of an orthopedic service that I would have the opportunity to build myself. I didn't know how far along they were in their search, but Silen had clearly sounded serious. I didn't for a moment think this might be one of those all-too-common situations where an African American physician was included as a candidate for the sake of checking off a nondiscrimination box. If this did work out, there was no way I could turn it down.

When I went up to Boston to interview, there didn't seem much doubt that the search committee was doing its final vetting. I didn't know if there might be one or two others under consideration, but my talks with Silen and the other chiefs of Harvard's teaching hospitals, as well as with Mitchell Rabkin, Beth Israel's CEO, were extremely positive. After a number of interview visits I was fairly confident, and not long after the last one Silen called to formally offer me the job.

Leaving Yale wasn't easy. The medical school had been my home for most of a decade, in essence for my entire academic career. To say that I appreciated the opportunities Yale had given me to grow and develop as a surgeon would be a significant understatement. Wayne Southwick had mentored me and nurtured my progress. He had become a dear friend as well as a teacher. I had close friendships with other colleagues as well, and being part of the Yale medical science community had always been so immensely stimulating. Beyond that, Manohar and I had built the biomechanics laboratory from the ground up. I knew that parting from that, and from him, would be a wrenching experience. But the offer to run my own department at Harvard wasn't one I could turn down, and so at the end of the semester I closed down my office, said my good-byes, and left for Boston.

It took a while for us to find a house in the Boston area— Anita and I had been married for several years, and two beautiful daughters had joined our family, Alissa and Atina (our third, Annica, would come along two years later). But at Beth Israel I hit the ground running. Near the top of my agenda was getting a biomechanics laboratory started. The obvious person for that job was Manohar, who during his seven years at Yale had established himself as an international leader in the field. I pulled out the stops to persuade him to join me, which meant that I quickly found myself in a friendly tug-of-war with Wayne Southwick. Wayne was at least as motivated to keep Manohar as I was to take him with me. If Manohar deserted along with me, the Yale biomechanics program would be in serious trouble. And in the end Wayne was able to dig a little deeper than I was, so Manohar stayed on at Yale.

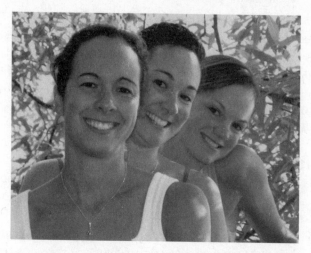

My daughters. Left to right: Alissa, Atina, Annica. Stockholm, Sweden, 2006. Photo: Thomas Ottemo.

My good fortune was that I was able to lure Wilson "Toby" Hayes, a bioengineering professor from the University of Pennsylvania. Toby Hayes came with a well-deserved international reputation as a brilliant and innovative scientist. He also turned out to be a skilled teacher and administrator, and under his leadership the laboratory quickly grew into one of the world's leading research facilities for orthopedic biomechanics.

With Toby attracting top students and the orthopedics department producing high-level research papers and increasing its clinical reach, we were definitely in the game—by which I mean the collegial yet highly competitive dynamics among Harvard's major teaching hospitals. These institutions were cousins, but there are kissing cousins and fighting cousins; as often as not these hospitals were fighting cousins.

Massachusetts General, Brigham and Women's, and Boston Children's, together with Beth Israel, constituted the Harvard Combined Orthopedics Program. Our challenge at Beth Israel was that each of the other hospitals had at least three generations of household name luminaries gracing their orthopedic departments, including the current chairmen: Henry Mankin at Mass General, John Hall at Children's, and Clement Sledge at Brigham's, Henry being the first among equals. Meanwhile, I was starting more or less from ground zero. Beth Israel had a small group of excellent orthopedic surgeons on staff but no academic activity and no teaching. I was the new young guy on the block, intruding into space that powerful old chiefs had long ago divided up among themselves.

All the churning went on once a month in executive committee meetings held at the Harvard Club's McIntyre Room, which looked exactly like what you'd expect of a Harvard Club meeting room—the wood paneling, the Persian carpet, the austere dignity. I was aware that I was entering treacherous waters. The rivalries, especially between Mass General and the Brigham, were deep and often fierce. But I got involved fast; there wasn't any alternative. In a short time I became close friends with some of my colleagues on the executive committee, who included Melvin Glimcher, a world-renowned scientist and senior professor at Children's. But friendly or not, I was glad for the boxing lessons I had picked up in my earlier years.

Just as at Yale, the selection of interns and residents was a regular bone of contention, except that at Harvard four departments were vying, not just a few individual professors. And there was no question that my presence stirred the pot, since now the executive committee had a member who was pushing strongly for minority candidates. In this endeavor I didn't exactly have any open and avowed enemies; I think everyone recognized that we were still badly lacking in diversity. But though I might not have had outright enemies, I did have opposition. And since I wasn't reticent, I did generate more than a little blowback.

At Harvard, again as at Yale, admissions had gone in certain directions because of the priorities of the individuals making the decisions. None of the eminent professors on the executive committee was racist, even my one persistent opponent, presumably. But prior to my arrival, the issue of diversity was not prominent on anyone's radar scope, so it didn't enter into admissions discussions the way it did after I came on board. Bias against minorities was, in that way, built into the culture. My job, as I saw it, was not simply to argue for one black applicant or another. It was to assert the need for diversity as an institutional desideratum—which I did to the utmost of my ability.

My strongest ally on the diversity front was Henry Mankin, the MGH chief and the combined residency program's director. But Henry had an array of formidable issues to deal with, and, like Wayne Southwick, he had only so much political capital. So he'd try to get me to lay back a bit. I'd be in the middle of making some point loud and clear, and Henry would lean over and whisper in my ear, "Gus, no. Not now, okay? Please." Sometimes he wouldn't even say anything, he'd just kick me under the table.

There was little diversity at that time among either residents or faculty. This was in the seventies, and even today the Harvard Medical School is woefully short on African American faculty. But socially, Boston was another story altogether, as different from New Haven as it could be. In Boston I was plunged into a mélange of cultures, some of them highly exotic, at least to me.

Nothing in my previous life prepared me for the Tavern Club, the immensely genteel haunt of Boston Brahmins and others whose status was only a rung or two beneath that level—many of them Harvard connected. The members list included Cabots, Lodges, Lowells, Saltonstalls, Holmeses, and Peabodys. Maybe if I had gone to Andover or Deerfield instead of Mt. Hermon I would have been more familiar with the high Yankee culture the Tavern Club epitomized. As it was, I felt at first as if I had entered a museum where an older, more aristocratic way of life had been preserved. The furnishings were elegant antiques. Everything about the club spoke of reserve and understatement, mixed with an unmistakable air of privilege and elitism. The kind of wit and wisdom that was daily fare at the Tavern Club wasn't like anything I had encountered elsewhere. I was happy to be there, though I wasn't quite sure that I belonged.

There was, as far as I could make out, only one other African American member. This was the Reverend Peter Gomes, Harvard's chaplain and an internationally known professor of divinity. There were no women. There had never been any women.

That very issue was raised at the first meeting I attended. During the discussion I leaned over and asked the member next to me if it would be appropriate for me to say something. "Of course," he whispered back. "Longevity has nothing to do with the right to speak." With that encouragement I threw caution to the wind and gave a brief speech about how women should have the same chance as men for the companionship and social enjoyment that Tavern Club membership afforded. A week later I was having lunch at the club when an extremely senior member sat down at my table and started harrumphing. "Dr. White," he harrumphed, "good to have you with us. But perhaps it would be advisable to get to know fellow members before being so forward in articulation."

The Boulé (Sigma Pi Phi, to give it its formal name) wasn't any kind of black Tavern Club, though there were certain parallels. The Boulé is the hundred-plus-year-old, national African American fraternal organization composed of men who have attained a certain level of accomplishment. To give you some idea, Martin Luther King, Arthur Ashe, Douglas Wilder, and perhaps 90 percent of the country's African American mayors are members, as are professionals and leaders from every field. The Boulé was the first African American fraternity, and over the years it spread out from Philadelphia (where it was founded by four doctors) to other large cities. When I was at Yale, New Haven had no Boulé chapter. Boston did, though. I enjoyed the Tavern Club immensely, with its lectures, poetry readings, and theatrical performances. But there I was an outsider who had been taken inside. With the Boulé I was an insider on the inside. At the Boulé dinners, dances, lectures, and family picnics I never had to think twice about being too forward in my articulation. There I was at home with my brothers.

There weren't that many Swedes in New Haven either, but Boston seemed to be full of them. For the first time in her American life Anita had a community of countrymen and women around, which delighted her. Actually, Boston's Swedes were a well-organized community, with a school, a home for the elderly, and a thriving chapter of SWEA, an international cultural/educational women's organization. I got used to hearing Swedish spoken around our house. Our children went to Swedish school. Anita became a leading member of SWEA and later served as president for several years. We went to dinners where they served salmon and potatoes with dill sauce, or meatballs and potatoes, or herring and potatoes, with strong coffee and apple cake for dessert. We listened to Swedish dinnertime speeches and sang Swedish drinking songs. We went to Sweden for our vacations. I might not have been native born, but I considered myself at the very least an honorary Swede.

Then there was Beth Israel, which was founded early in the twentieth century by Jewish doctors who back then were not permitted to practice at Mass General or the other major area hospitals. Of course, the hospital wasn't all Jewish; in fact its charter stated that it was founded to serve all races, creeds, and colors. But Beth Israel's president was Jewish and so were most of the department heads and many of the staff physicians. My new home was a Jewish institution where I was surrounded by Jewish colleagues. I went to bar and bat mitzvahs, I ate Jewish food, Anita and I were invited to Passover seders. I began to understand what several thousand years of history meant to the Jewish people, much of it having been spent as despised outsiders. I had great admiration for the way they had endured so much and overcome so much. No question that Jews had a claim to be called soul people, at least Jewish soul people.

You could say that in Boston I was swimming in diversity, appreciating it and enjoying it, and, if I thought about it, congratulating myself on my luck. I'm sure my good fortune had an impact later on, when I came to think about diversity in a larger, social sense. But meanwhile there was the medical school, where diversity was still a source of tension. There was also Brown University, where I had been a trustee for four years and was now on the Board of Fellows. And Brown was experiencing some disturbing racial problems.

As a fellow, I stayed attuned to goings-on at Brown, but I wasn't part of its daily life. I didn't have an intimate familiarity with the problems, except it was clear that minority students, specifically black students, weren't happy. They felt they weren't being treated properly, that their needs weren't being addressed. There was a background to this. In 1975 there had been a black students' strike. Later there had been a building takeover and protests of different sorts, some of them recent. There was obviously a lot of frustration and general discontent. For its part, the administration was doing its best to deal with events as they happened, in an ad hoc way. From what I could see, the school cared about its minority students—it just did not know what to do about them.

From somewhere the idea dawned on me that the university ought to be taking a proactive approach to its racial difficulties, not just responding to brushfires. When I was a student at Brown, thirty years earlier, there had been only fifteen or twenty African American undergraduates altogether. Now there were more than that in each class. Back then the concept of integration had been a lodestar. But though the school had embraced that ideal and had made strong efforts to attract students of color, something had obviously broken down. Integration—the idea that minority students could and would somehow naturally assimilate into the majority culture—had clearly not worked. Why not? And what approach might make for a better, more harmonious relationship between the black students, their white classmates, and the university community as a whole?

I didn't have an answer to that, but I did think that for the sake of its health the university should be trying to find what that answer might be. With that thought in mind, I went to Brown's president, Howard Swearer, with a proposal. The most recent racial protest had been resolved, I said, the community had pretty much put it in the past. But now that we were in a period of calm, wouldn't it make sense to put together a group of people from outside the school to look at the problem as a whole? Outsiders would be less emotional, they wouldn't have vested interests. No one would be fighting for power within the university; no one would be seen as biased or self-aggrandizing. The group could be made up of people with experience and wisdom on the issue of minorities in American life and especially minorities and educational institutions. Call the group a visiting committee. Give them access to any information they want, let them speak to everyone they need to. Charge them to study Brown and come up with recommendations for how to address the issue of race on an ethnically diverse campus in the way most beneficial to the entire university community.

Howard Swearer listened carefully as I outlined the idea. He thought about it, but not for very long. I was sure the problem had been fairly high up on his list of concerns for some time. "Yes," he said. "That sounds like it makes a lot of sense. Let me give it some consideration. I'll get back to you shortly."

When we next sat down, Swearer knew how he wanted to proceed. "Gus," he said, "it's a good idea. I'd like to ask you to establish a committee along the lines you mentioned. And I'd like you to chair it."

I wasn't terribly surprised to hear this; I knew Swearer to be a serious and thoughtful person. But I was thrilled by it. And as we talked further I got even more excited by what he was asking of me—and especially by what he was *not* asking of me. Swearer wasn't laying down any guidelines. He wasn't telling me who he thought should be on the committee or what the procedures might be or what kind of recommendations he was looking for. He had decided to open the university up to the scrutiny of outsiders. He was giving me free rein. He was acting with a lot of implicit trust and, I thought, considerable courage.

As it turned out, I was able to attract some true wisdom to the committee. Kenneth Clark, the psychologist and civil rights activist, accepted my invitation; as did Louis Sullivan, founder of the Morehouse school of medicine and later secretary of health and human services in the G. H. W. Bush administration; Jim Comer, my old psychiatrist friend and colleague from Yale; and Ron Takaki, the eminent Japanese American professor of ethnic studies at Berkeley. Other equally thoughtful people joined us as well. Ten months and a great deal of work later, including three multiday full-committee visits to the university, we presented to the Brown Corporation a report entitled "The American University and the Pluralist Ideal." The seventeen of us on the committee had talked with more or less every distinct group in the university, from faculty and administrators and alumni to parents and cafeteria workers and security guards and athletic staff. We had opened ourselves up to student groups and individual students, to minorities and nonminorities. We heard from blacks, Asians, and Latinos about their anxieties and insecurities. We solicited input from every corner.

The committee focused on minority life, on what steps Brown could take to create a more welcoming environment, so that minority students would feel that they were equal and valued members of the community and so that the school would recognize their distinctiveness and appreciate the enrichment they brought to the life of the university. In the end we presented the corporation with seventeen recommendations, all but one of which was adopted. We recommended that Brown should increase its minority numbers among students and faculty. We recommended that minority students be encouraged to form clubs and other organizations that would provide an avenue for the expression of their cultural identities. We urged the university to broaden its course offerings on ethnicity-related subjects and to expand the functions of the Third World Center, a student union whose activities catered to minorities, many of whom traced their heritage back to so-called Third World countries.

Our primary goal was to move Brown beyond diversity per se. When we interviewed Charles Baldwin, Brown's chaplain, he emphasized that the ideal we were working toward was pluralism. Diversity meant that the university community would include people of different races, ethnicities, religions, and so on. To a certain extent Brown had achieved diversity. Pluralism moved beyond diversity in that it conceived of a community where minorities were not simply present, but where they were welcomed, where their cultures were acknowledged and valued. That is, a community where minorities would not be expected to be subsumed by the majority culture, but where they would take their own distinct places at the communal table.

I felt these recommendations, taken as a whole, would be a major step forward in improving minority life at Brown. Because we had listened attentively to so many of the university's different groups, our recommendations in effect mirrored attitudes and thinking that were current in the school community. We were in essence articulating and giving shape to opinions that had already taken hold, which was why the university corporation so enthusiastically welcomed the road map we outlined. "The Visiting Committee report was," President Swearer wrote, "a most significant contribution and its influence will be felt for many years at the University."

The Brown visiting committee report was a watershed in the university's history of race relations. But it turned out to be far more than that, at least as I saw it. As we moved along in the process, I realized with increasing clarity that while we believed our recommendations would be significant in and of themselves, on a deeper level we were looking for a change in the university's fundamental identity, its sense of what it was and what it should be.

From its inception Brown had been an unorthodox place. In earlier times the Rhode Island colony had been notorious as a haven for the disaffected and disenfranchised. Founded in 1764, Brown (originally the College of Rhode Island) was, as its charter put it, "liberal and catholic," that is, it welcomed the disaffected and different-thinking. Diversity then had mainly meant diverse religious groups, including not just religious minorities but even freethinkers. But in the post–civil rights era the idea of diversity had broadened considerably. In particular, it now prominently included racial and ethnic minorities. At bottom what we, the visiting committee, were saying, was that it was time for the university to embrace diversity as something more than an interesting part of its history. It was time to institutionalize diversity and its correlate, pluralism, as an institutional ideal. We were asking Brown to make diversity into one of the pillars of its fundamental identity.

We did not simply think that our recommendations would improve minority life, we believed they would create a richer community altogether, in line with the richer, more textured community the entire country was becoming. That was how the university could best produce graduates who were "duly qualified for discharging the offices of life with usefulness and reputation," as the charter so succinctly defined Brown's ultimate goal. This was an ongoing aspiration, we felt.

After the Brown visiting committee experience, my life at Harvard and Beth Israel didn't change outwardly. I was in the clinic and operating room almost every day, doing my best to diagnose and treat spinal problems. I taught. I wrote a book for back pain sufferers—*Your Aching Back*. I continued to build Beth Israel's orthopedic service and help shape the Harvard combined program. But at the same time I found myself thinking more and more about diversity, about the place of African Americans in medicine and the role they—we—played in delivering health care.

In 1994 I had the chance to put some of my thoughts in order when the National Medical Association's orthopedic section asked me to deliver that year's Orthopedic Scholars' Lecture. I was working at the time on spondylotic myelopathy, degenerative changes in the aging cervical spine, so my first thought was to discuss my findings in that area. But I was also concerned about the state of blacks in orthopedics. Orthopedic residencies were always highly competitive, and at that time the situation in medicine was worsening regarding payments to doctors and hospitals. In addition, the national projections were decreasing considerably for the number of orthopedic surgeons that would be needed in the future. All this meant that the number of training slots was likely to be cut back. And this inevitably meant that the small number of African American trainees was sure to shrink even further.

I flashed back for a moment to my first meeting with Montague Cobb at his club in Washington, that time I had returned briefly from Vietnam. "We've opened up a hole in the line," he had told me. "Now we have to get as many people as possible through

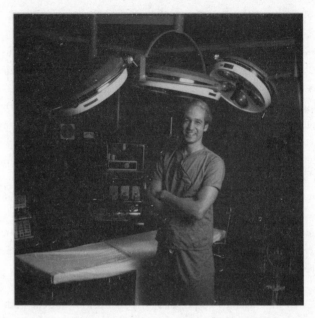

Orthopaedic Surgeon-in-Chief, Beth Israel Hospital Operating Suite, 1987. Photo by Richard A. Chase, © 1987 by the President and Fellows of Harvard College.

before it closes back up." From statistics I was reading and from the high anxiety I was sensing from medical students interested in pursuing orthopedics, most especially from black students, I could see the hole beginning to close. So when I sat down to compose the Scholars' Lecture I thought, No, they hear about bones and joints every day of the week. This is the time my black orthopedic brothers and I ought to be focusing on our profession, what's happening to our place in it, and what we ought to do about it.

With that I wrote out what was essentially a journey through my own career in orthopedics, and what I'd seen along the way in terms of our progress and our problems. I talked about the difficulties African Americans have when it comes to networking, that is, in leveraging our contacts for our mutual benefit. I talked about the legacy of the colonialized mentality and the stereotyped images of ourselves that do so much harm. I emphasized how crucial it is that we take part in the national orthopedic associations, that we work hard on committees and subcommittees, that we do everything we can to reach positions of visibility and influence. These are our institutions, I said; we need to claim our ownership rights in them through our involvement. We have to counteract our disadvantages by working the system as vigorously as we are able in order to help ourselves and each other. We can't allow our numbers to dwindle and watch while we turn into dinosaurs—for our sake, and even more for our patients' sake. Studies show, I told them, that blacks receive inferior health care as compared to whites. Racism is still rampant, overtly and covertly. At least some of the disparity is due to the relative scarcity of minority doctors. We need a lot more African American physicians, not fewer.

We need to integrate ourselves into the mainstream in a more powerful way. We have to persuade the profession that the issue of diversity is a priority, not just some sort of peripheral concern that interests a few individuals but leaves most unmoved.

I'm not sure to what extent my remarks might have affected my audience. But after the lecture, as people were milling around and leaving, Timothy Stephens took me aside. Stephens was chairman of the orthopedic section. "Gus," he said, "I don't know how serious you might be about this. I hope you are. I don't have a budget for it, but I could at least support some teleconferencing if you want to try to get something started."

Over the following week or so I got on the phone with Stephens and a number of other orthopedists from the meeting who I knew shared my views: Charlie Epps, James Hill, Ray Pierce, Tony Rankin, and Randall Morgan. Over the next several months we decided on two courses of action. The first was to take the diversity issue to the top level of the American Academy of Orthopedic Surgeons. We'd lay out our concerns with them and see if we couldn't set up some procedures or mechanisms that would at least begin to address the scarcity and lack of visibility of minority orthopedic doctors. With that decided, we contacted Dr. William Tipton, the Academy's executive director, and set up a meeting.

We had no idea what Tipton's response might be, whether he would be adversarial or sympathetic, whether we'd find ourselves involved in a discussion or a negotiation or a collaboration or what. Our own mind-set was not to be confrontational, but to be strong advocates for the need for minority doctors and diversity in the profession. We were ready to make our case, in a friendly manner, but directly.

We held the meeting in the Red Carpet Club room at Chicago's O'Hare Airport. The Academy's executive offices were in Rosemont, very near O'Hare, and since those of us attending were coming from all points in the compass, Chicago was more or less a central location. As it turned out, Bill Tipton wasn't adversarial at all. On the contrary, he seemed to see the sense in what we were saying. It was obvious that this wasn't the first time in his life he had heard the word diversity and that he had thought about it himself.

While we talked, I was thinking about how different this was from my confrontation with Charles Womer, the CEO at Yale–New Haven Hospital. There I had felt I was punching uphill against a hostile opponent. Here we were trading thoughts rather than punches in a respectful atmosphere. Tipton's bottom line was: I understand what you're saying, fellows. We have to address some of these things. I'll be back in touch.

When Tipton got back, it was to put us together with Doug Jackson, the incoming president of the Academy of Orthopedic Surgeons. Jackson was a sports medicine specialist from Long Beach, California. In his practice he took care of various high school football teams, which included many black athletes and Samoans along with white players. Vietnamese and Cambodian refugees had flocked to Long Beach, and they were his patients too. Jackson had given a lot of thought to issues of diversity and the need for minority doctors. Like Bill Tipton, he believed something needed to be done. He was ready to work with us. Why not set up an ad hoc committee, he said, to decide how best to move forward.

The ad hoc committee consisted of himself, Tony Rankin, and Clarence Shields. Tony was a professor of clinical orthopedics at Howard, and Clarence a prominent African American surgeon in Los Angeles whose practice included the NFL's Los Angeles Rams and the UCLA football program. Both men were creative thinkers with real insight into the problems of minorities and health care. A couple of weeks later they called me with news that the Academy had decided to establish a formal committee on diversity. They asked if I might want to chair it.

I couldn't have asked for a more promising outcome. An AAOS committee on diversity meant that the place of minorities in health care would become an institutional matter, recognized, in orthopedics at least, as a core issue. A formal committee would work to eliminate barriers to minorities entering the specialty and would address other problems of minority health care—and those efforts would become agenda items for the Academy at large. This would be a major step in making concerns that had mainly been visible to minority doctors visible to all.

Beyond establishing a committee, Doug Jackson took other initiatives. Over time these resulted in Ray Pierce becoming the official Academy representative to the National Medical Association, where there had never before been a formal connection. Another of our original colleagues, Richard Grant, was appointed to the certifying board for orthopedic surgeons, the first African American to serve in that essential capacity. Then Tony Rankin and later Alvin Crawford (my old friend from Memphis, the one who integrated the University of Tennessee Medical School) were named to the Academy's board of directors, the first time African Americans had been in that position too. Eventually, Tony Rankin became president of the Academy himself.

These appointments, in addition to the new AAOS diversity committee, did wonders to raise awareness among orthopedists generally. I felt as if we were finally achieving recognition, not just for who we ourselves were—the fact was that everyone involved in that initial O'Hare meeting had already achieved a level of prominence—

but for the issues we represented. Formally embracing diversity signaled that the orthopedists, at least, were moving to deinstitutionalize the racism embedded in their corner of the medical world. It demonstrated, too, that they were serious about taking on the pervasive problem of disparities in health care.

All this happened in the mid- and late 1990s, thirty years after I started looking for a residency and was told by my friend Bobbie Dibble to get serious, that other than two or three individuals at Howard and Harlem Hospital there were, literally, no African American orthopedic surgeons in the entire country. Now we had a strong core of accomplished, board-certified specialists, individuals who could take their places confidently in the profession's highest positions.

Our initiative with Bill Tipton and Doug Jackson had borne fruit. But during those early teleconferences, our original gang of seven had decided on a second course of action as well. The National Medical Association, the black AMA, had an orthopedic section. But there was no separate association of black orthopedists that might be capable of representing its issues within the AAOS. Establishing that kind of association or society, independent but affiliated with the Academy, would give us an effective platform for sharing concerns and research both among ourselves and with the larger orthopedic community.

We already had a step up in that direction. For quite a few years, Charles Epps, one of the true African American orthopedic pioneers, ran a Howard/Meharry orthopedic alumni gathering, which those of us who weren't Howard or Meharry alums also attended. Charlie Epps was like an elder brother to us all. Everyone looked forward to our annual luncheons with him and the opportunity to get together for discussion and advice with friends and colleagues.

That luncheon group was a springboard for the society we wanted to form. After some discussion, we decided to name ourselves the J. Robert Gladden Orthopedic Society. In 1949 J. Robert Gladden had been the first board-certified African American orthopedic surgeon and the first elected to membership in the American

Academy of Orthopedic Surgeons. He had died at the age of fifty-eight in 1969. There wasn't a living black orthopedic surgeon who didn't think of him as our great predecessor.

We had plenty of models for the Gladden Society. Quite a few other societies had formed under the umbrella of the Academy, including the Cervical Spine Research Society, of which I had been president one year, and the Ruth Jackson Society—the association of women orthopedists. Each of these separate societies had its independent membership, its dues, its mission. But they were all housed together with the Academy's offices, so communication with the Academy and with each other was excellent. And operating as part of the Academy, each society had a chance to teach, to present its materials, to be included in the Academy's programs. The Gladden Society would be another building block in our effort to institutionalize diversity in the orthopedic world. Because we would be part of the Academy, I thought of it as a significant evolutionary step in reshaping what had been until relatively recently an exclusively white, male culture.

As we got closer to formalizing our plans, we touched base with the Ruth Jackson Society and cranked out a constitution and bylaws. The Ruth Jackson Society was for women, a small minority of orthopedists. The Gladden Society would be pluralist, for minorities of all kinds, though African American in origin. Our goal would be to share research, to educate, to increase diversity in the profession, and to work toward eliminating ethnic disparities in the care of musculoskeletal health problems. We even hoped—as Lou Sullivan said in his keynote speech to our first yearly meeting—that we would influence other medical specialty societies to establish similar groups.

By the late 1990s perceptions of disparities in health care were growing, both among doctors and in the public generally. A number of eye-opening studies had been done comparing health care received by minorities and by whites. Even controlling for socioeconomic factors, researchers were finding significant differences in treatment and outcomes. In some areas poorer-quality care was leading not only to inferior outcomes generally but to higher mortality rates. Racial and ethnic differences were showing up in cardiology, gynecology, oncology, ophthalmology, psychiatry, orthopedics—right down the line, in one specialty after another.

I knew about these findings, and I thought that this endemic and unacceptable situation should be a major focus of the Gladden Society and the new AAOS diversity committee. But one event in particular triggered a different kind of understanding for me.

I had boarded a plane back to Boston from Chicago, where I had been attending an AAOS meeting. Ordinarily I used traveling time to catch up on reading journal articles or reports, so I tried to keep as much to myself as I could. On that trip, though, an attractive young woman sat down next to me. I was already reading something, but she had said "excuse me," and I had gotten up to let her into her seat. She looked to be college age, dressed neatly, very polite, and, it turned out, very talkative. Pretty soon she had me involved in a conversation.

She had just graduated, she told me. But actually, she was just coming back from a convention she had been to.

"Oh," I said. "What kind of convention?"

"A tattoo convention," she said. "I'm a tattoo model."

I instantly found myself looking for tattoos, as inconspicuously as I could, not that she didn't notice. There was nothing on her hands or her face, nothing on her neck as far as I could see.

"You can't see anything because I'm wearing a high collar, long sleeves, and slacks," she said. "Other than my face and hands, my entire body is one hundred percent covered."

I was a little taken aback. I'd seen plenty of tattoos, but 100 percent body coverage was something else. I'm sure I had forgotten most of the lectures I heard in medical school, but one that stood out vividly had been about tattoos and the diseases tattooing can transmit. The professor had shown spectacular slides of people with tattooed arms, tattooed backs, and one or two of people whose entire torsos were covered. The individuals who tend to have these tattoos, the professor said, were sailors, prostitutes, and circus sideshow people. Also convicted criminals. There were three diseases in particular that are associated with tattoos, he told us: syphilis, tuberculosis, and leprosy.[1]

The idea we got from the lecture was that these individuals, these sailors and prostitutes and carnival people, weren't quite in their right minds, or at least they weren't quite normal. There was something subrational about people who would choose to do this thing that carried the danger of syphilis, tuberculosis, and leprosy. I don't think the professor actually said anything explicitly negative. But he didn't have to. The sense that hovered over all this was that these folks were maybe not quite everything they could be. Not really up to the level of normal people—like those of us in the lecture hall.

But my traveling companion was clearly neither a sailor nor a prostitute. Nor was she a sideshow person or a convict. She was vivacious and intelligent; she seemed normal in every way. She told me she had majored in English literature. As we talked, it somehow came out that I was a physician. But as soon as I said that, she got quiet and a kind of sad, forlorn look came over her face. "I hate to go to doctors," she said in a whisper, as if she were talking half to me, half to herself.

"Well, I guess I don't blame you," I said. "Nobody really enjoys going to doctors. But why do you say that?"

"Because they treat me so badly," she said.

I saw it instantly. She didn't have to say another word. I pictured her sitting in a doctor's office unclothed for an examination. I could just see the stares, the amazement, the intrusive questions, the doctor maybe inviting one or two others in to take a look. "Can you believe this? Come in here, get a look at this." And how would the doctor treat her? Would he look at her as a curiosity? Would he be standoffish, maybe a little uncomfortable? Would he try to hide his distaste for what he was seeing? Would he look at her as a little less than a full human being? He almost surely would approach her with something other than simple objectivity and compassion for whatever it was that was troubling her.

I had actually seen that kind of thing more than once. Not with tattooed people, but with obese people and elderly people. I knew doctors who did not relate to these patients as they should have, who were a little put off or impatient, who weren't as attentive as they would have been with someone more supposedly "normal." There was nothing particularly strange about it. People have their likes and dislikes, and doctors are no different. But I always found it a little troubling, hearing that kind of thing from colleagues.

That night I was thinking over my talk with the tattooed young woman and suddenly something clicked. To the doctors she saw, this girl was "other." Maybe with full-body tattoos she was more dramatically "other" than many who also didn't fit the norm— racially or ethnically or culturally. But essentially she was the same as they were, "other" in a way that would inevitably trigger reactions from doctors that were neither sympathetic nor especially compassionate. And those visceral reactions were very likely to affect the medical care they provided. They might be a little less engaged, a little more rushed. They might be more likely to allow stereotypes to enter into their judgments. You didn't have to be an overt racist or bigot of some sort for this to happen—like that surgeon back at the Crump Hospital in Memphis who had killed Mrs. Dixon. It would be enough to have feelings of distaste or discomfort, even feelings you might not acknowledge to yourself, or maybe weren't even explicitly aware of. No doubt some of the disparities that were being identified were due to outright prejudice, but the chances were good that most had a far less obvious origin, and that the origin was likely to be found in the emotional ways doctors responded to the individuals they were treating.

When I got back to work the next morning I went to see Dr. Dan Goodenough. Dan was a cell biology professor. He was also master of the Oliver Wendell Holmes Society, one of the educational associations to which Harvard assigned each medical student. I felt as if I had had a revelation. "Dan," I said, "exactly what are we doing about health disparities?"

9

DIAGNOSIS AND TREATMENT:
THE SUBCONSCIOUS AT WORK

Emotions are . . . the function where mind and body most closely and mysteriously interact.

—Ronald de Sousa

Patients and loved ones swim together with physicians in a sea of feelings. Each needs to keep an eye on a neutral shore where flags are planted to warn of treacherous emotional currents.

—Jerome Groopman

MY REVELATION WAS, in a sense, a commonplace. My airplane encounter brought home to me the truth that medical care is a human interaction. Emotion enters into it, feelings that are overt and others that may be hidden or unacknowledged. Liking and disliking play an obvious role.

Professors Debra Roter of Johns Hopkins and Judith Hall of Northwestern are among the country's leading experts on this subject. Medical care, they show in their various studies, is a two-way street. Physicians bring to the doctor-patient relationship their scientific expertise and clinical experience; patients bring their knowledge of themselves, their instincts, the circumstances of their lives, their histories. "Communication," according to Roter and Hall, is "the fundamental instrument by which the doctor-patient relationship is crafted and by which therapeutic goals are achieved." It has a profound effect on medical outcomes because it gives the physician the necessary context for a full understanding of the patient's symptoms.[1] Communication is most effective when there is an "open relationship" between doctor and patient. But that kind of relationship requires respect and rapport. When there is discomfort or dislike on the doctor's side, it can and very often does negatively affect clinical thinking and conclusions.

Doctors are not dispassionate scientists, making definitive decisions solely on the basis of test results and impersonal diagnostic algorithms. Medicine, as Lou Sullivan says, is the delivery of scientific knowledge and expertise given in a social context. The human part of the health-care equation is essential to providing the best treatment. And it's that human part that draws on ingrained beliefs and judgments, on our prejudices and our stereotypes of those who are different from us. The human part encompasses our likes and dislikes. The tattooed young woman drove home for me what kind of impact the doctor's perception of the patient can have. And that allowed me to draw the connection between the physicians' inner disposition toward those they are treating and the profoundly disturbing disparities in care that more and more studies were showing. After that I felt I had been called to action.

I wanted to talk to Dan Goodenough because as master of the Oliver Wendell Holmes Society he was responsible for the educational training of a large segment of Harvard's medical students. What I didn't know was that Dan Goodenough had had his own revelations and that he was working hard to put those revelations to use in educating his students.

Dan is an internationally known Harvard cell biologist, a gentle person and elegant researcher who specializes in tracing the complex pathways by which cells communicate with each other, and whose other major concerns include human health and global environmental change. His students perennially consider him one of the best teachers at Harvard Medical School, not only because of his lucid presentations but because his personal warmth seems to naturally engage them. Dan is a person whose humanity is written on his face. His commitment to students and teaching is, I think, every bit as deep as his commitment to laboratory science.

I didn't know it, but when I went to see Dan he was incubating in private what turned out to be a highly innovative course for students and faculty in self-awareness as an essential element in the work doctors do.

His own revelation, what he now describes as "a precipitating moment," was the birth of his second daughter. "The umbilical cord was wrapped around the baby's neck," he says, remembering back. "Her fetal heart rate began to fall and they had to do an emergency cesarean. It worked out well. The baby was delivered in time. My wife didn't die. But it was a humbling experience. If it had been a hundred years ago or if we had been living in a Third World country, they probably would have both died."[2]

But that wasn't the end of the story. A week later Goodenough's wife, Carol, developed a raging fever and had to be rushed to the hospital. It turned out that during the cesarean a highly resistant streptococcal infection had gotten into her system. Goodenough watched while the doctors struggled unsuccessfully to stem the infection. Days passed as Carol's condition grew steadily more critical. And as it did, her physicians became increasingly anxious and desperate.

"The handling of this emergency was pretty badly done on a lot of levels," Goodenough says. "I watched how the physicians who were attending to her were unable to communicate with each other. They were angry with each other and writing and rewriting over each other's notes—to the point where the nurses didn't know what they were supposed to do. It was very chaotic.

"And in all the chaos they missed a very simple diagnosis, which was that thrombi were developing and throwing clots to her lungs. The doctors were coming in every day and giving her one excruciatingly painful pelvic exam after another. They were concentrating on that and didn't notice that her hands and feet were swelling and that she was having difficulty breathing. Things that any physician in a different context would have observed right away and would have been very concerned about."

But the doctors did not notice. They were too focused on finding the source of the infection and on their frantic search for an effective antibiotic therapy. Ten days or so after she was admitted, with the doctors still concentrating on her inflamed pelvis, Carol Goodenough went into heart failure. It was only then, at the eleventh hour, that anticoagulants were administered and she was pulled back from the edge of death.

The trauma of watching his wife go through this impressed itself powerfully on Goodenough. But the lessons he drew from what had happened went beyond those a layman would have drawn. Goodenough was a worried husband experiencing the fear and anxiety of watching his wife almost die, but he was also a young medical school professor teaching first- and second-year students. "Here were all these wonderful young people coming in," he says. "I was seeing them at the beginning of their journey toward becoming doctors. And then, as my wife was going through this, I was interacting with doctors on the other end, after they had emerged from their training. Something had clearly gone wrong. And whatever it was presumably had to do with something in—or not in—their medical education."

Dan Goodenough's revelations from this experience, his "precipitating moments," were two. First, he saw what a powerful and potentially deadly effect physicians' emotions could have on the clarity of their judgment. He had no doubt that if the doctors who were dealing with his wife had been discussing a case that was going well, over lunch in the cafeteria, they would have communicated easily. But in a highly stressful situation, where nobody knew what was going on and they were in danger of losing their patient, their emotions kicked into high gear. And that kept them from stepping back and looking at the case anew, with more objective eyes, which would have revealed to them what they had missed.

That was one lesson he took away from how his wife's near-fatal infection was treated. The second had to do with how he himself was treated during the many anxiety-ridden days it took for her illness to be resolved. "During the crisis," he says, "I felt like I was totally invisible. No one would look at me, no one wanted to talk to me. It was a new experience—complete invisibility.

"I knew something about that from things I had read or heard, about handicapped people often feeling that way, as if they were ignored and treated as if they didn't really exist. I had heard more about it regarding African Americans. There was even a famous book by the great black writer Ralph Ellison entitled *The Invisible Man*. But this was the first time I had ever experienced such a thing myself. Here I was, a perfectly normal white male person, deeply involved in my wife's illness, and *I* was invisible."

How was it that the physicians couldn't communicate well? And why was it that they assiduously ignored him, even though he was white, male, unhandicapped, and a medical school assistant professor to boot (though he hadn't told them that, and this wasn't a Harvard hospital)? If they were treating *him* that way, he thought, how would they treat others who might have even less claim on their attention—women, or blacks, or non-English-speakers?

In Goodenough's mind, the problems these experiences illuminated had a single root. Emotions—fear, anxiety, aversion—had imposed themselves on what the doctors were doing. They got in the way of treatment and they got in the way of decent human interaction. He began thinking that medical schools should find a way to teach students to be aware of how emotions affect the cognitive functions by which doctors diagnose and treat—and no less important, how emotion affects their perceptions of others, most especially those who are different from themselves.

"I see it as the same problem," he says today. "The fundamental flaw is the lack of self-awareness. What are you feeling in a particular situation? Why are you feeling that? How do those feelings get in your way, and how can you get your own affect out of the equation and be an open, curious, connected person, rather than an angry, scared, close-minded one?" Thinking about the same problem, Pat Croskerry, a medical school professor and emergency physician in

Canada put it succinctly. "When our viscera are involved," he says, "we do not make good judgments."[3]

Croskerry argues that while clinical decisions should be made objectively, in practice that most often does not happen. Doctors, he says, "develop both positive and negative feelings toward patients, which may impact on decision quality."[4] That same insight provides a good deal of the steam for Jerome Groopman's examination of the kinds of errors doctors make when they confront a medical problem. Groopman is a colleague of mine at Harvard who realized at some point that even though he was trained in a top medical school, had decades of clinical experience as a cancer specialist, and is a teacher of many years standing, he had never really considered why things go right in medical thinking and why they go wrong. When he started asking his colleagues that question, he found that few of them had answers either.

This is the question he explores in his wonderful book *How Doctors Think*. "I long believed," he writes, "that the errors we made in medicine were largely technical ones . . . But as a growing body of research shows, technical errors account for only a small fraction of our incorrect diagnoses and treatments. Most errors are mistakes in thinking. And part of what causes these cognitive errors is our inner feelings, feelings we do not readily admit to and often don't even recognize."[5] Cognition and emotion, Groopman insists, are inseparable.[6]

Groopman's assertion of the interrelationship of cognition and emotion isn't simply the inductive conclusion of a physician-writer based on his own and others' experiences of treating patients. There is a neurobiological explanation for why our reasoning function is interwoven with our feelings. Various neuroscientists, philosophers, and psychobiologists have made convincing cases for that proposition, the best known of whom may be Antonio Damasio, a professor of neuroscience and director of the Brain and Creativity Institute at the University of Southern California.[7]

In his seminal book *Descartes' Error*, Damasio spells out how the mind with its cognitive functions has evolved from the body and its emotional systems and how they function together through neuro-networks that connect the mechanisms of feeling with the brain's decision-making centers. "Feelings," he says "come first in development and retain a primacy that pervades our mental life." They "constitute a frame of reference" and "have a say on how the rest of the brain and cognition go about their business. Their influence is immense."[8]

Damasio is not looking specifically at the problems of medical diagnosis and how doctors feel about their patients, but his exposition has great relevance for the way bias influences treatment and outcomes. He points out too that states of feeling often impinge on reasoning in covert, unrecognized ways. "While the hidden machinery underneath [cognition] has been activated, our consciousness will never know it ... [T]riggering activity from neurotransmitter nuclei ... can bias cognitive processes in a covert manner and thus influence the reasoning and decision-making mode."[9] Researchers looking into the effect of prejudice and stereotyping on the delivery of medical care have noted exactly this phenomenon. Overt biases—racism, sexism, ageism, and the other isms—are obvious in their consequences for health care. But the impact of unintentional bias and unrecognized stereotyping can be just as, or even more, adverse.[10]

Dan Goodenough's revelatory experiences started him thinking about creating a special course for Harvard's medical students and faculty. As he read through the growing literature on the relationship of emotion to medical decision making, he began to focus more specifically on how conscious and unconscious attitudes—biases, prejudice, and stereotyping—contribute to treatment errors and health-care disparities. The key, he thought, was to center students' attention on the need for self-awareness, especially self-awareness regarding the students' own cultural identification and how that affects their attitudes toward other groups.

While I was talking to Dan about what role the Oliver Wendell Holmes Society might play in educating students about these issues, I was drawing some conclusions from my own past. I had, through pure good fortune, never personally experienced the worst of what racism can do. But I certainly had had my own experiences of negative stereotyping—from my childhood in Memphis to some of my fellow docs in Vietnam for whom a black surgeon just did not fit into their mental categories.

What I had experienced from them was an attitude of disregard rather than what I would call out-and-out stereotyping. But I had good friends with more vivid stories. There was, for instance, my friend Harris Gibson, MD. Harris is a thoracic surgeon who practices in the suburbs of Boston. Harris got his medical training at Meharry and did residencies in general surgery and thoracic surgery with the Public Health Service. He was for a while president of the Middlesex East District Massachusetts Medical Society. Even today there are not many African American surgeons in Boston, and when Harris was younger there were hardly any, especially in the suburban hospitals where he was affiliated. He was laboring out there for years all by himself.

One day Harris was seeing patients in one of these suburban hospitals, a place where he had just started working a short time earlier and wasn't known well. He was on the surgical recovery floor, looking in on his patients, moving from one patient's room to the nursing station and back to another room in his usual brisk and determined fashion. Harris isn't just a first-rate surgeon, he's a surgeon's surgeon. He's also a serious man who doesn't waste time. But while he was making notes at the nurse's station, he sensed that someone was watching him. It was the charge nurse. Harris didn't know her, but she seemed none too friendly. In fact she seemed to be giving off vibes of suspicion, as if she wasn't sure what this so-called doctor was doing on her floor, or even if he was a doctor. She reminded Harris of Nurse Ratched from *One Flew over the Cuckoo's Nest*.

After watching him for a while going back and forth from patients' rooms to the nursing station, she finally made up her mind. She had to confront this obvious imposter. "Uh huh," she said loudly, so the other nurses and doctors in the nurses' station would notice what was happening. Near six feet tall, she towered over him. "Tell me, exactly which doctor are you?"

Harris looked up from his writing. He stood up and smiled warmly at her. He knew exactly what she was thinking. "I?" he said, just as loudly. "Oh. I'se de witch doctah." Nurse Ratched retreated fast. A few of the personnel in the station ran off somewhere smothering their laughter. Others just smiled, shook their heads, and continued with what they were doing. But from that moment the incident entered into the lore of that hospital and several other suburban hospitals, to where the story quickly spread. Nurses and doctors talk about it to this day.

Stereotyping, of course, isn't usually so humorous. David Schneider is a psychology professor at Rice University and an acknowledged expert on how stereotyping functions as one of the mechanisms in our cognitive toolbox. "Stereotypes," he says, "are generalizations with deep resonances in our mental lives and profound consequences for our social behavior."[11] Prejudice, which is so often the outer manifestation of mental stereotyping, is, he says, "the set of affective reactions we have toward people as a function of their category memberships."[12] That is, our emotional predispositions toward people we see as "other" can and do have real-life consequences. In the world of health care, those consequences pertain to diagnosis and treatment.

Lay people have a well-known tendency to look up to doctors. Doctors are our resort when we fall ill or injure ourselves, and often they can heal us, ameliorate our suffering, or even save our lives. Doctors have special expertise and professional wisdom. They are caregivers, humanitarians by definition. Yet doctors are as guilty of stereotyping and the prejudice that flows from it as other people. Those prejudices show up in the hospital and office where patients are exposed to them, and in the medical school, where students are.

One way Harvard tries to bring stereotypes and prejudices to light and counteract them is by making it possible for students, faculty, and staff to report incidents anonymously in the *Focus,* a newsletter that goes out to the schools of medicine, dentistry, and public health. The medical school's Multicultural Fellows Society had been collecting these sorts of reports for a number of years, and when I became the Holmes Society master the newsletter picked up my suggestion that they should be published so the entire community could make use of them. I considered them an institutional mechanism for helping to change behavior. They provided an outlet for emotions that might otherwise stay bottled up, a chance for the larger community to become aware of problems, and an opportunity for instigators to reflect on what constitutes unacceptable behavior.

The short descriptions are printed, followed by a comment or response, usually by a professor. Here is one of these student "Incident Reports."

"One night in the emergency room, the residents began joking about a homosexual patient, laughing about 'this faggot.' Seeing the look on my face the chief resident asked whether I was gay. I replied that I was not but that I have plenty of friends who were. The group laughed. Then they changed the subject, laughing at the morbid obesity of a patient they had seen that day. 'Oh, sorry,' the chief resident chuckled while facing me. 'Do you have friends who are fat?'"

And here's part of the response, by a professor of psychiatry.

"When medical students speak about negative experiences during clerkships, they often mention disparaging remarks made about patients. While such behavior is offensive in any context, it is especially troubling to future physicians ... Put downs of the vulnerable have long been part of the medical culture. Students have always picked up this 'informal curriculum' in corridors and lunchrooms ... But in recent decades ... a new kind of professional authenticity has broken with the convention of 'double entry' patient-doctor communication, a perverse etiquette that had us thinking we could respect patients at the bedside while speaking disrespectfully of them in private."[13]

Here's another incident report.

"I was the only woman on a medical team. Everyone knows how important it is for a team to 'bond,' often through a shared sense of humor. Unfortunately, I found this humor frequently involved oohing and aahing at attractive nurses. These jokes made me feel alienated from my team, especially when one intern jokingly commented that he wanted to take one nurse into a back room and 'slap her around some.'"

And here's the response by a female pediatrician and social medicine instructor.

"Gender-based discrimination pervades the practice of medicine in insidious ways. It is insidious because on the surface, dramatic changes have occurred for women in medicine. Twenty years ago women made up less than a third of incoming students. H[arvard] M[edical] S[chool] had no formal sexual harassment policy; women's health as an area for research and practice was barely recognized; and only a small portion of senior faculty were women. [But] while times have changed, our students continue to report multiple examples of sexism."[14]

These and many similar incident reports point out the persistence of derogation of "out groups," women, gays, elderly, Hispanics, blacks. They and the "responses" also demonstrate that we are in the midst of a changing medical culture. Students, faculty, nurses, staff doctors—all these groups have become far more diverse than they used to be. As a result, the attitudes and stereotyping that were commonplace for years are less and less the norm. Where many colleagues are women, African American, Hispanic, or gay, manifestations of prejudice aren't simply considered an unremarkable part of life, as they once were. They are noted and elicit disapproval. They begin to fade out of the realm of those attitudes that make up society's norms and into the category of those that most people find obnoxious and unacceptable.

But these sorts of changes in social mores take years, even generations. The subordination of women and the abhorrence of homosexuality are deeply ingrained historical phenomena, as is, of course, racial prejudice. These are not uniquely American phenomena, but they are writ large here—perhaps because they are so outrageously out of keeping with our expressed ideals.

In 2001, at the same time Dan Goodenough was developing his course and I myself was considering how to counteract these prejudices among medical students and doctors, Congress was growing increasingly alarmed by just how pervasive and destructive disparities in the delivery of health care seemed to be. As a result it charged the Institute of Medicine with assessing the problem of racial and other prejudices. The book that came out of this charge, *Unequal Treatment,* shocked the medical world into recognition of what was going on.[15] Many of the studies the book adduced were hard to believe, though no less true for that. Others that came afterward pounded home the lesson of how deep our problems were and how urgent the need was to find some way of addressing them.

10

HEALTH-CARE DISPARITIES: RACE

Of all the forms of inequality, injustice in health is the most shocking and inhumane.

—Martin Luther King, Jr.

UNEQUAL TREATMENT revealed an underside of American health care that most doctors had no idea existed. Here we are, the book announced, at the start of the twenty-first century, four decades after the civil rights laws were passed, and the medical world is riddled with prejudice and discrimination. The question was: How could this possibly be?

In clear, dispassionate prose, *Unequal Treatment* spelled out the extent of the problem. African Americans and Hispanic Americans received poorer care than whites right across the board. Since the charge from Congress to the Institute of Medicine was to look at racial and ethnic disparities, the researchers and writers also examined the more limited number of studies regarding Asian Americans, Native Americans, and Pacific Islanders. Of the various racial and ethnic minorities, though, African Americans were, for various reasons, by far the most thoroughly scrutinized.

Given the long history in America of racial prejudice, it wasn't a surprise that blacks were especially subject to inferior treatment. Compared with whites, they had lower rates of cardiac surgeries, fewer hip and knee replacements, fewer kidney and liver transplants. Diabetic blacks were more often amputated than diabetic whites. Non-diabetic blacks were amputated more often too. Blacks were more likely to receive open surgeries rather than the less dangerous laparoscopic procedures. Surgeons didn't operate on them as often for equally operable lung cancers. They received less pain medication for the same injuries and diseases. They were more likely to be castrated as a treatment for prostate cancer. Black infant mortality was almost two and a half times that of white babies. The overall black mortality rate was 60 percent higher than the white rate. African American males in Harlem, one study concluded, had less of a chance of reaching age sixty-five than males in Bangladesh.[1]

I knew about most of these and similar findings from my research for the Shands lecture to the Academy a year and a half before *Unequal Treatment* came out. But to many doctors, hearing such things came as a rude awakening. I think it's a truism that most physicians try to give all their patients the best care they can. So the suggestion that the profession as a whole might be prejudiced against African Americans or Hispanics strikes most doctors who aren't focused on social issues as frustrating and inexplicable. For people with full and hectic schedules, laboring under insurer-driven financial pressures and inundated with important new biomedical findings they need to keep up on, discrimination isn't high on the list of concerns. It's kind of a nonproblem, something that doesn't involve them. Discrimination may exist, but someone else must be doing it. Or else there are large social forces at work that they, as doctors, have no control over; poverty and education, for example. Of course, impoverished and poorly educated people will probably receive less-optimal care. That's, unfortunately, the nature of the system—hardly a reflection on doctors themselves.

But *Unequal Treatment* drew on a decade and more of studies. And these studies had become increasingly sophisticated. In particular, many of them controlled for variables, including the effects of socioeconomic factors, education, disease severity, and access to treatment. It might be a commonplace that poor people often didn't have private doctors, that lack of insurance meant it wasn't easy for them to see specialists, that they might not be able to afford medications. But why was it, then, that black cardiac patients in the same hospitals and with the same insurance as white cardiac patients received less catheterization, less angioplasty, less bypass surgery? They were even less likely to receive common heart disease medications such as beta blockers, anticlotting drugs, or aspirin.[2] Why was it that, in one of the country's top teaching and research hospitals, black emergency room patients were more likely to be referred to doctors who were still in training as residents while whites were more likely to be referred to experienced staff specialists?[3] And, in my own field, just why in the world was it that African Americans brought into ERs with long bone fractures were less likely to receive opioids and other analgesics?[4]

Pain is universally interesting precisely because it's universal. Everybody has pain sometimes and some people have pain frequently or even chronically. We've all had conversations where we've talked about what kinds of pains we have and how badly we've suffered from them. There's even a kind of general curiosity as to what the worst pains are. Kidney stone sufferers often swear that the pain of passing such things is above and beyond. Acute sciatica has its strong advocates for most painful, as do migraine headaches. But childbirth can hardly be relegated to second place behind anything, though root canal infections also make most pains pale by comparison. I'm not sure exactly where long bone fractures fit into the hierarchy, but they are, without a doubt, exceptionally painful.

Let's imagine that a person—black or white, it doesn't matter; the physiology is exactly the same—is wheeled into a busy emergency room with a broken tibia, maybe from a bad fall. The tibia, or shinbone, connects the knee with the ankle bones. It's the larger and stronger of the two bones of the lower leg. It takes considerable force to break a tibia. But when it is broken, here's what happens.

The tibia, like all bones, is encased in a thin sheath of tissue called the periosteum. The periosteum itself has two layers. The outer one is richly endowed with blood vessels and what are called nociceptive nerves, that is, nerves that transmit pain. The blow that broke our patient's tibia undoubtedly caused tissue damage in the region, and the broken bone ripped open its periosteum sheath. Maybe it did this in one place, if the patient has a simple fracture.

But it could have happened in several places. Tibia fractures also frequently involve damage or fracture to the fibula—the thinner and weaker of the two lower leg bones. The broken bone ends can be sharp, and the wound may have left splinters or spikes of bone. If a surgeon isn't careful, a sharp bone end can penetrate right through her surgical gloves.[5]

But even if the bone ends are not sharp, they'll move around and jiggle any fragments or spikes. The torn periosteum, with its many pain-sensing nerves, will be flooding the brain with pain signals, and any additional movement will aggravate the nociceptors further, creating more pain. In addition, the periosteum's broken blood vessels will be bleeding into the area, and the pooling blood may pressure and irritate the surrounding muscles and other tissues, magnifying the pain even more.

All that may happen even if EMTs have splinted our patient, immobilizing the bone to a certain extent. If they haven't done that for some reason, every movement, the joggling of the gurney or transferring our patient to an X-ray table, for example, will cause excruciating pain.

All that pain has a reason, of course. It's the body's way of telling the brain in no uncertain terms not to move the injured limb. The brain has to keep things as still as possible down there. Only that way will healing begin and new bone matter be laid down to start fusing the break. That message has to be very loud and very clear, which explains why the pain volume is so high.

Now, here's what happens once our patient is in the ER. Let's assume it's a big, busy city hospital—which is where the main analgesia studies were done. With all the activity, it may take a while for a nurse to do an assessment and triage the new arrival. A fracture patient who isn't in shock, whose blood pressure is not down, and who is not bleeding profusely won't be at the top of the triage, but he will be urgent. Everyone knows the level of pain here. But still, it will take some time for one of the ER docs to get around to him. If the break is so bad he needs surgery, he'll be medicated and up he'll go to the operating room. Otherwise, his leg will be immobilized in a large brace or cast and he'll be fitted for crutches. And regularly, if that patient is black, he'll be given less pain medication than his white fellow human being. Not infrequently, he'll get no pain medication at all.

That, by the way, is true for Hispanic as well as African American patients. In fact, the groundbreaking analgesic study of this sort was done on Hispanic fracture patients.[6] I'm discussing African American disparities first because, even though I readily understood that other groups were also subjected to disparate health care in equally serious and meaningful ways, as a black physician my own experiences and thinking were initially focused on race issues. Also, because the racial divide is so exemplary of implicit prejudice, understanding how that works may be a key to unlocking the way prejudice works vis-à-vis other minorities. In any event, the bone fracture researchers were so impressed by their findings that they repeated their Hispanic study in a different city with black patients. After that, other researchers were sufficiently taken by those results that they began looking into postoperative analgesic prescriptions and found large disparities there as well.[7]

While most attuned doctors were disturbed by all of the *Unequal Treatment* disparity revelations—on cardiac care, transplants, surgical procedures, and others—to me, as an orthopedic surgeon, it was the long bone breaks that really stood out. A bone break is about as simple and straightforward as an injury can get. It has no relation to culture or language or unhealthy lifestyle, or whether African Americans might be adverse to some kinds of treatments. It simply must be fixed, and the considerable pain of it has to be addressed. Broken bones and analgesia are an ideal case to test whether the health-care delivery system is functioning in an egalitarian way, as we expect it to. And the health-care delivery system failed that test miserably. As Professor Jack Geiger wrote in *Unequal Treatment* after surveying the spectrum of health-care disparities, bone-break cases are "particularly troubling."[8]

If you try to get at why this particular disparity happens, several explanations suggest themselves. One is the historical assumption that blacks do not experience pain the same way whites do. They have, as one nineteenth-century medical account put it, "an insensibility of the nerves." Endowed with a more primitive, robust resistance to pain, African Americans don't actually need as much pain medication as whites. Of course, this is utter nonsense, and nobody today would ever get up in a lecture and state such a thing. But it stands out in the historical literature. That belief became part of the culture of medicine at some level, and it's still out there in the background ambience. Then there's the conscious or unconscious assumption that African Americans coming into the ER may be drug addicts, or at least may be seeking drugs. That is to say, you'd better be especially careful with narcotics when you're dealing with black patients.

There's another background assumption at work too. An African American psychiatrist, talking about his white colleagues at a major West Coast teaching hospital, said, "I knew a lot of white psychiatrists who thought it was a truism that all black people were angry with whites, that all of their black patients were angry and mistrusting."[9] Irving Allen, another African American psychiatrist in the Boston area, talks to black patients about how to survive in a medical setting. "Be cool," he tells them. "Be extremely careful not to appear hostile." But the fact is that patients in severe pain are often scared and angry. And doctors aren't different from other people, despite all their training. Confronted with what they perceive as anger or dislike, especially black anger, they will tend to back off, or at least not engage as they would otherwise. The doctor's response might be, "I don't really want to deal with this. Let me get this cast on and get on with somebody else." And that too might impinge on prescribing the appropriate pain medications.

All this is aside from just plain old subconscious or maybe even conscious prejudice. But even without these stereotypes and assumptions—blacks don't feel as much pain, they might be addicts or drug dealers, they might be hostile—doctors will sometimes simply let things slip, especially in the rush of a busy ER. That happens vis-à-vis white patients too. Pain management often just isn't handled as well as it should be. But for African Americans it happens a great deal more often.

DR. ALVIN POUSSAINT has a long memory. A preeminent African American psychiatrist, Poussaint has been on the faculty at Harvard since the late 1960s. He is prominent not just as a therapist but as an administrator who has made an art of providing counsel and support for students of every racial and class background. Poussaint is an internationally sought-after speaker and consultant who served as the adviser for *The Cosby Show* (where Bill Cosby played a doctor, though not a psychiatrist). For years he's been a leading voice on children's mental health issues. Recently he and Cosby coauthored the widely read *Come On, People,* aimed at the difficulties faced by African American young men and their parents.

Poussaint operates out of a small, cluttered office in a Harvard-affiliated children's center. He comes across as anything but the high-profile, friend-of-Cosby, best-selling, international luminary that he is. Soft-spoken and avuncular, he engages easily with visitors, but in a reserved, cool way. When he talks about some of his experiences with America's segregated health system, his even tones belie the shameful nature of the history he is recounting.

Disparities in health care have been on the national agenda since the 1990s, and *Unequal Treatment* put the subject front and center for the medical establishment in 2003. But Poussaint has been thinking about these issues far longer. Growing up in East Harlem in the 1930s and 1940s, he remembers that African Americans from his neighborhood who needed to be hospitalized almost always ended up at Harlem Hospital. He had a visiting professorship at Harlem Hospital in the 1980s. At that point it was a well-run hospital that was providing an excellent level of care, with dedicated doctors and bright trainees. In the earlier part of the century, though, its reputation was different.

Back then it was notorious for atrocious overcrowding and decrepit, inadequate facilities. Poussaint remembers people joking that if you ever went in there, you'd never come out alive. "As a result," he says, "a lot of people who were sick were not going to go to Harlem Hospital. They were going to delay or postpone—they were going to have to be half dead before they'd seek care." Mt. Sinai, which was only five blocks away, was considered a white hospital, not welcoming to blacks. The same was true for New York's other major private hospitals such as Columbia Presbyterian and New York Hospital. African Americans and Latinos were shunted to the municipal hospitals instead.

The same system of de facto hospital segregation was in place in most northern cities. Montague Cobb called it "The Negro Medical Ghetto." Seriously inferior care was a fact of African American life everywhere above the Mason-Dixon Line. In the South it was a great deal worse. Southern segregation, as Poussaint points out, was set up to value white lives and devalue black lives. Medical care was an especially egregious aspect of that devaluation of black lives. Through most of the region, hospitals were segregated by law. White hospitals wouldn't allow blacks in no matter how desperately ill or injured they might be. "Colored" hospitals were few and far between and utterly deficient in terms of services and care at all levels.

In 1964, though, the civil rights laws made hospital segregation illegal. The following year Poussaint was in Jackson, Mississippi, as the southern field director of the Medical Committee for Human Rights. His job there was to provide medical care for the civil rights workers and to help integrate the hospitals—which were all still segregated a year after the law passed. Resistance was fierce. Black doctors found it impossible to get admitting privileges for their patients. In Mississippi and Alabama, where Poussaint was mainly working, antiblack racism had an iron grip on people's minds. "When they [hospital officials] talked about desegregating the hospitals they would talk about how blacks had terrible body odor. They smelled bad and had greasy, dirty hair that would mess up all the linen. And who would want to be in a room with them?" For the two years he was there, Poussaint found himself up against pathological, visceral-level hatred.

After that he came to Boston, first to Tufts University, then to Harvard. Boston's hospitals were integrated, but that didn't mean they had been bled of racial antipathy. "I remember when I first came to Boston," he recalls, "there was all this racism here. A lot of the ancillary staff [at hospitals] were from south Boston or Dorchester, who had very negative feelings about black people, who were later part of the anti-busing effort, and just used the n-word all the time. When they had face-to-face contact with black patients, the patients picked up instantly that they were not welcome and they were not liked."

In the South, negative stereotypes of African Americans permeated black-white interactions. That was true in the North also. But why did they run so deep? And why were they so persistent?

Research in social cognition gives us some of the answers. David Schneider, the Rice professor of psychology, is only one of the many experts who point out that categorization is fundamental to the way our minds work. Categorization is perhaps *the* major organizing principle that allows us to sort through and make sense of the world's overwhelming fullness and variety. He and his fellow psychologists talk about two basic category types, nonsocial and social. Nonsocial categories have to do with how we divide and understand the world of things. Social categories have to do with how we divide and understand the world of people.

Of the social categories, three, according to Schneider, are important enough to be called primary. These are gender, race, and age.[10] That is to say, we recognize these divisions immediately, without the need for conscious thought. It takes time and familiarity before we are able to place someone in a religious category, to classify her as Jewish, Christian, or Muslim. But we recognize gender, race, and age automatically.

There are several reasons why we do. Gender, race, and age are almost always unmistakable visually—they are "perceptually salient." They are also rooted physically and biologically. Schneider suggests that these categories have evolutionary significance as well. Gender is a reproductive marker, age a marker for experience and wisdom, race an in-group/out-group (potential friend/potential enemy) marker. Each of these categories indicates attributes that were of fundamental importance for our ancestors' survival.

Primary categories are deeply embedded. Gender and race, social cognition researchers tell us, are among the first human categories children learn to distinguish—before the age of two, and without anyone having to teach them. Such primary categorization, says Schneider, is "hard, if not impossible to inhibit."[11]

Stereotyping is a corollary of categorization. Stereotyping fixes on various features our minds associate with the category in an inflexible way (the root of the word means solid or hard). Stereotypes incline us away from differentiating individuals from types. And while stereotypes can be either positive or negative, social cognition psychologists tell us that whites have a strong tendency to think of African Americans in terms of negative attributes.[12]

How does all this go toward explaining how it is that fair-minded, compassionate doctors end up giving less pain medication to blacks than to whites for equally painful conditions? More bluntly, why do they allow African Americans to suffer more?

The answer is that categorization and stereotyping are such elemental mechanisms of cognition that we can't get away from them, with racial identification being one of the primary classifications. And since in white minds blacks are more associated with negative attributes, that perception gets incorporated into "normal" patterns of understanding.

Because these things happen subconsciously—they are automatic mental processes—it's no wonder that bias may be implicit and unrecognized, yet shows up starkly in medical practice. In the course of interviewing health-care professionals for a study of disparate care, Harvard medical anthropologist Mary-Jo Good talked with an African American attending psychiatrist who told her that "in his consultations on psychotropic medications he often finds that primary care physicians prescribe less current drugs for their black patients. When he asks them why, they are baffled and unaware."[13] But you don't have to be a medical anthropologist or statistical researcher to notice the phenomenon. Here's a student Incident Report from the *Focus* newsletter: "During team rounds the resident referred to a black patient by her first name, removed her bedclothes, and examined her abdomen and breasts without drawing the curtain in a two-bed room. The next patient, [a white woman] who was called Mrs. Jones, underwent the same examination while she was carefully draped, and the curtains round her bed were drawn."[14] Why are those white doctors treating their black patients differently? They do not know. They do it without thinking.

Stereotyping is like a mental conduit that channels people away from considering those in out-groups as individuals. Other large forces that have the same effect come into play too. In this regard, medical anthropologist Good has focused attention on the culture of medicine itself. She has been especially interested in the way the medical world trains doctors to recognize disease.

Good, who has been studying this subject for several decades, uses the term "medical gaze" to convey the essence of her assessment. By "medical gaze," she and other social scientists mean the culture of medicine that conditions physicians to focus on the patient's physiological symptoms and biomedical indications and discourages them from taking into account the social context. As students, she says, doctors learn to value "what medicine cares about" and to discount the human side. Time pressures, the stresses of the work environment, and the need to see many patients all reinforce the expedience of this so-called prescriptive approach to treatment.[15] Another leading teacher and researcher puts it this way: "Doctors are taught that their own personal background, and the characteristics of the patient . . . should be excluded from consideration in the formulation of clinical decisions."[16]

Students learn this approach from their professors and supervisors, whom they emulate, and from the structure of the medical school curriculum. Many students are attracted to caring for the poor or working to alleviate minority health problems. But these kinds of humanitarian projects tend to become less important as they move on to clinical work in their third and fourth years and into their internships, where they are faced with making hard therapeutic decisions with potentially grave consequences.[17]

Operating from within this biomedical perspective, doctors find certain kinds of patients harder to treat. Patients may have problems that are exacerbated by their social circumstances, that get in the way of medical therapies. Patients may not comply with doctors' wishes and expectations. They may indulge in high-risk behaviors that obviate therapies. Patients of this sort throw doctors off from providing the care they have learned is most effective. Giving them optimal care requires exploration and insight into their individual lives, which physicians may not be able, or willing, to give and are not, in any case, trained to do. Such patients are frustrating and time consuming in a medical environment that more and more demands efficiency. All this feeds into doctors' attitudes toward those they treat.

The kinds of patients who bring these sorts of extramedical problems into their interactions with doctors tend to be more poorly educated and from lower socioeconomic groups. They also tend to be from racial and ethnic minorities. Over time, many doctors build or buy into stereotypes of these groups in ways that can and do influence diagnosis and treatment. One influential study that looked at physicians' perceptions of patients showed that doctors thought of African American patients as less intelligent, less educated, more likely to be drug abusers, less likely to follow doctors' orders, and less likely to enjoy the help and support of others while in treatment than their white patients—*even though the study was controlled for education level, income, and other potentially confounding factors.* Finally, white doctors felt less affiliation—that is, less friendliness—toward their black patients.[18]

What we see from almost everyone who has studied disparate care is that the causes are multidimensional. Some are overt and clear: low socioeconomic and educational levels, for example. Other causes are subtle, operating below the level of consciousness. Doctors bring perspectives into the medical equation that are, as Good points out, deeply conditioned and rarely examined. Stereotypes—negative stereotypes when it comes to race—are at work all the time whether we want them to be or not.

One present-day consequence of our long history of racial inequality and conflict has to do with the "friendliness" item that was part of the study I referred to just now. The authors asked doctors which patients they could see themselves being friends with. More white doctors answered that they would be likely to be friends with white rather than black patients. It's hardly a surprise, then, when other researchers tell us that African Americans find themselves having more communication problems with their white doctors and feel more disrespect from them. Or that African Americans have more trust in African American doctors and derive higher satisfaction from their visits with them.[19] Alvin Poussaint treated many black and white patients over a long career. His African American patients, he says, "always wanted to feel a connection with me as another black person."

My own experience over an equally long career treating both black and white patients was a little different. I'm not sure how many of my African American patients were looking to make a connection with me as another black person. But I was always aware of trying to make a connection with them. Like Poussaint, I may have leaned over backward to make absolutely sure they knew I was concerned for them personally and would do everything in my power to take care of them—in part because I was mindful that they may well have experienced a different attitude in other medical settings. I was also, I think, instinctively attempting at some level to ascertain: Is this a person who feels his or her black identity? Or is this person aloof and distant from it? I don't make judgments of African Americans on the basis of how "black" they are. Each of us has his or her own mechanisms of dealing with the fact of being black in a white society. But the answer did mean something to me emotionally. Did I share something deep in my own sense of identity with this person, or did I not?

For better or worse, black identity is a strong definer for African Americans, in a way that white identity is not for whites. At the courses in culturally competent health care that we have developed at Harvard, which I'll be talking about in Chapter 12, we ask participants how often they think about their race each day. There's a spectrum of answers, from "all the time," to "occasionally," to "never." It's only the white participants who answer "never." Tim Wise is a teacher and activist on racism. He writes in his book *White Like Me* about an exercise in which black people and white people are asked to list the things they like about being black or white. Black people always come up with a list of positive cultural attributes. My own list would include, for example, camaraderie, music, fortitude, tight friendships, athleticism, achievement in the face of obstacles, and "soul," among others. White people, when asked the question, find it difficult to respond at all. Race is simply not an identity for them as it is for blacks.

Because black identity is a bonding mechanism for African Americans, it's quite understandable that they might feel less comfortable, at least initially, with white than with black physicians. But since most African Americans are treated by white doctors, that feeling can have negative effects. It's something that inevitably impacts communication, and despite all the ultrasophisticated technology and biomedical advances of today's medicine, patient-doctor communication is still, as Jerome Groopman puts it, "the bedrock of clinical practice."

For doctors, communication is central to figuring out what's causing the problem your patient has so you can treat it properly. Effective communication not only enables the doctor's understanding, it affects the outcome of the treatment he prescribes. When doctors and patients talk to each other effectively, patient compliance with therapies is better, outcomes of treatment are better, and patient satisfaction is better. This is true from depression to diabetes to hypertension to cancer treatment, even for joint replacement outcomes. And for communication to work best it has to be reciprocal. That's critical. It's not just the way the doctor talks and listens to the patient, it's the way the patient talks and listens to the doctor.

We've already seen some of the negatives that go into doctors' orientation toward patients of color. Those negatives impact communication for the worse. Studies show that white doctors spend less time talking with black patients than they do with whites, and they do so with less empathy. In addition there's the paternalism that has historically characterized doctors' relationships with patients of all types, which magnifies the problem substantially. "Many physicians," says Dr. Bruce Siegel, a health policy professor at George Washington University, "are trained to think of ourselves as little gods."[20] The doctor-as-God business may be an exaggeration, but it's not that much of one. There have always been entrenched power-status relationships in medicine between patients and doctors. And minority status, being black or Latino, means that you're down there at the butt end of the hierarchy.

But it's not just the docs. African American patients bring their own baggage with them to the medical encounter. They do tend to feel less comfort and less satisfaction with white doctors. That's partly an affiliation factor, as we've seen. But there's a lot more going on than that. There's a history here that most white Americans may be only vaguely aware of, but that is ingrained somewhere in the consciousness of almost every African American.

One aspect of that history is the long and truly terrible story of the medical establishment's use of unconsenting and often unaware black subjects for medical experiments. Generally speaking, public knowledge of this subject is limited to the infamous Tuskegee Syphilis Study, but that was just one instance in a plethora of inhumane, often outrageous, experiments. The dark record of these things is conveyed in Harriet Washington's book *Medical Apartheid*. The phenomenon touched enough black individuals and groups over a long enough period that it helped create in the black community as a whole, she says, a deep distrust and fear of what doctors might do to you.[21]

This fear—Washington calls it "black *iatrophobia*"—is not an ancient subject, interesting only as an historical curiosity. Its legacy is very much with us today. Here's Dr. Poussaint again, reflecting on his different experiences with white and black patients: "I frequently knew that many of my black patients were highly suspicious and very uncomfortable with the techniques that psychiatrists use. They felt threatened . . . their experience with psychiatrists historically was that they heard somebody saw a psychiatrist and the next thing you knew he ended up at a state hospital." His black patients, he says, needed a high level of reassurance. "They needed to know that I was interested in them as a person, not just as a subject for analysis, not just that I was looking for psychopathology. My therapy with black patients was much more personalized and interactive."

In other words, even this African American doctor's black patients needed exactly the kind of psychosocial, personal engagement that is markedly missing from so many doctor-patient interactions— most especially between white doctors and black patients.

Medical experiments using vulnerable and unsuspecting black subjects were, of course, only one element in the centuries-long devaluation of black life in America that had—no surprise here—a powerful impact on African American psychology. One consequence was the "colonialized mentality," Frantz Fanon's phrase for the condition in which suppressed peoples come to identify with their suppressors and adopt the suppressors' view of themselves. The most vivid expression of this state of mind I've seen is in an autobiographical remark by the great Nigerian novelist Chinua Achebe, describing his racial perspective as a young man. "I did not see myself as an African to begin with. The white man was good and reasonable and intelligent and courageous. The savages arrayed against him were sinister and stupid or, at most, cunning. I hated their guts."[22]

Self-hatred like this is extreme, but feelings of inferiority and lack of confidence vis-à-vis the white world are anything but. The common black feeling of being slighted, disregarded, and stereotyped led Ralph Ellison to endow the protagonist of his well known book with the illusion that he was, simply, invisible. He existed, but the world around him didn't see him, or certainly did not see him for who he was. That kind of psychodynamic is common enough among African Americans so that the psychologist Franklin Anderson terms it "the invisibility syndrome."

We see related, if less disruptive, feelings of insignificance all too frequently among black male students at Harvard Medical School. These are young people who basically can walk on water. They're gifted, intelligent, articulate. They should be flying, hitting on all cylinders. But too many of them will have a profound lack of self-confidence. It's perplexing to me. I want to sit them down and say, What could possibly be wrong with you?

One young man of this sort came into my office. He was working on a PhD at MIT and going to medical school at the same time. He walked in and told me he wanted to be an orthopedic resident but he understood it was extremely difficult to get a slot. Did I think there was any possibility at all for him?

When I asked about his grades, he said he was getting all "high honors" at Harvard.

"How about MIT?"

"Pretty good," he said. "All As, one B."

I got up and shook hands with him. "Orthopedic residency?" I said. "Do you realize you are a national treasure?"[23]

This profound lack of self-confidence isn't the only black psychological syndrome we see. One of our African American residents had been an all-conference linebacker at a top football university. He looked the part, six two or so with huge, Mack-truck shoulders. He was also bright, insightful, well on his way to becoming a skilled surgeon. But on rounds or in meetings or simply in small group discussions you could hardly hear him, he was so unnaturally soft-spoken. The reason for his voice level and for his self-effacing demeanor? He was afraid of scaring white people. He knew the stereotype of the angry, violent black man well, and he was trying as hard as he could to distance himself from it.

The insecure MD/PhD student and the overcompensating football player are only two examples of the kind of African American adaptive behavior I've seen so often. At bottom, what it comes down to is discomfort with their white surroundings, a wariness and uncertainty about how they will be perceived—especially poignant to me because I lived through my own share of those feelings, always on the lookout, always with my radar tuned up. Erving Goffman, the sociologist who wrote *Stigma* and *The Presentation of Self in Everyday Life*, held that "the stigmatized individual may find he is unsure of how . . . normals will identify him and receive him . . . He has a sense of not knowing what others "really" feel about him."[24] Goffman wrote that forty-five years ago, but it is just as true today.

These are some of the feelings of inferiority and wariness that African Americans bring with them to the patient-doctor medical encounter, which is typically hierarchical in any event. These feelings may not be uppermost; they may be buried deep enough so that they aren't front and center in the patient's mind. But they are there. And they bear down on what goes on between themselves and their physicians.

In recent years the idea of patient-centered medicine has gained increasing traction among doctors. Incorporating patient input and considering patients as partners in their health care is an evolving counterweight to the prescriptive, "medical gaze" approach most physicians have been conditioned to. The Institute of Medicine, the Robert Wood Johnson Foundation, the Kellogg Foundation, the American Hospital Association, the American Academy of Orthopedic Surgeons, and other leading health-care organizations all have programs designed to increase patient engagement. These programs reflect the generally accepted understanding that effective communication involves patients equally with doctors. But the racial barriers to a more egalitarian concept of the doctor-patient relationship remain very high and very persistent.

The name of the game, of course, is outcomes. It is obvious that the more effectively patients can tell doctors about their problem, the more likely the doctor will be able to make a correct diagnosis. It's obvious, too, that the better the communication, the more the patient understands and trusts the doctor's recommendations and prescriptions, the more likely he or she will be to comply with them.

But there is also a less defined but powerful psychological factor at work. In my own practice I was always convinced that the emotional support I could give and the optimism I could convey had by themselves a strong effect on my patients' recovery and overall sense of well-being. I wanted my patients to be sure about my commitment to them, my desire to see them progress, and my conviction that they would. Although I never did any formal study, I was sure that this attitude made a difference. In the little book of aphorisms I kept in my head, one of the leading ones was: "Damn treatment. What are you going to do for your patient today?" Treatment after an orthopedic operation—the antibiotics (if they are necessary), the analgesics, the rehabilitation—are pretty much givens. But what else, in addition to my surgical care, was I going to be able to give my patient?

That "what else" had to do with the mind. We learn so little about the mind in medical school. And yet the mind has such immense influence on the body. What I was doing, or at least trying to do, was similar to giving my patients a placebo. I was stimulating their perception that they would get better.

It's the support, the caring of the doctor and the empowering of the patient, that is key, not only to effective communication but to releasing the uncharted power of the mind on the healing process. But nothing of that sort can happen if the black patient is not recognized as a full and equal person, of worth in her own right—if she does not find in the speech, the attitude, and the welcoming demeanor of her physician an acknowledgment of that simple fact.

The neuroscientist Antonio Damasio writes movingly of the physician's need to connect with the mind of the patient, so often full of concern and confusion. "It is of course true," he observes, "that all of the great physicians have been those men and women who are not only well versed in the hard-core physiopathology of their time, but are equally at ease . . . with the human heart in conflict."[25] The problems of race and medical disparities are not Damasio's concern, but he is nevertheless addressing what may well be the essence of the invidious effect of racism on the delivery of health care—the disconnect between the physician and the heart and mind of his patient. Assaulted on one side by denigration and stereotyping and on the other by the vulnerabilities of her own psyche, the heart of the African American in need of care is truly, as Damasio would put it, a human heart in conflict.

The medical community, I think, is slowly coming to understand how race affects what happens when doctors and patients talk. The question is: How do we increase that understanding?

IN 2001 I WAS SIXTY-FIVE YEARS OLD. I had been a practicing surgeon for thirty-five years. But now I could feel myself being drawn to the problem of unequal care like a moth to a flame. I had been involved in advocacy for black students for years. I had had that experience with minorities at Brown University. I had helped put diversity on the agenda of my fellow surgeons in the orthopedic academy. I felt somehow as if my whole life as a doctor was leading me to this point.

Not long after I began talking to Dan Goodenough about disparities in treatment, he stepped down as master of the Oliver Wendell Holmes Society. It was a stroke of fortune that as the search committee geared up to find a replacement, I got a call from the dean of medical education urging me to be a candidate. The master of the society was deeply involved in student education. He or she was also a member of all of Harvard Medical School's various standing committees. Being master, if that happened, would give me an opportunity to bring unequal care into the ongoing discussion of the medical school's concerns.

I was well aware by then that African Americans are not the only minority that experiences unequal treatment. Latinos do, women do, gays do, the elderly, Asian Americans, and others. The more I thought about being the Holmes Society master, the more excited I became. I wasn't sure exactly what I might do to help move Harvard toward grappling with this profound, society-wide problem. But I thought I could at least see a way to start it off.

11

HEALTH-CARE DISPARITIES: WOMEN, HISPANICS, ELDERLY, GAY

I don't know what's such a big deal about treating a human being like a human being.

—Dr. Joseph Kramer

THE HOLMES SOCIETY OPENING was fortuitous beyond anything I could have planned. I was sixty-five, just about the right age to move myself out of the operating room. I knew of more than one situation where surgeons had kept working longer than they should have. It's a hard, painful thing to quit doing something you've devoted your life to, and an extremely delicate situation for colleagues and hospitals—let alone patients—if your competence begins to deteriorate while you're still on the job. I had been involved in one situation like that myself as chief of service, and I knew of others. I was absolutely determined nothing like that was going to happen to me. I wanted to exit at the peak of my skills, while I was still providing the highest level of care I could and still getting as much enjoyment from surgery as I always had.

By the time I went into my last operation, I had heard from Dan Lowenstein, the dean of medical education, that the search committee had finalized my selection as master, which set off all sorts of ideas I had been nurturing for years about trying to provide students with certain ideals of patient care and humanitarian medical practice. Here was an opportunity to significantly contribute to the professional development of doctors in training. I had always loved working with students, and this would afford me a far higher volume of interaction than I had had before. Not least, as master of the Holmes Society I would have a platform to try to further the goals of diversity and equal care that had been consuming concerns for years now.

My farewell surgery was a lumbar spine herniated disk operation, something that a large number of back pain sufferers can relate to. Something I could relate to myself, not just as a surgeon, but as a patient, since I had had a similar procedure done several years earlier. In the operating room I paused for a moment at the side of my patient, already asleep and intubated. But I wasn't swept by any need to somehow mark the occasion. The nurse handed me the scalpel and I made the incision—the same way I had been taught to do incisions by Victor Richards and Don King a hundred years ago. Using the scalpel, I worked my way down toward the spine through the musculature and fascia, as I had done so many times before. I detached the yellow ligament that covers the protruding elements of the spine, and there it was: the disk—bulging out of its proper place between the vertebrae and pressing against the nerve root, usually whitish gray but now pink and inflamed from the pressure.

The surrounding vascular tissues were inflamed too, engorged and angry looking. This patient had been in severe pain, and no wonder. In my magnifying loupe the nerve looked as thick as a pencil, easy to see and easy to grasp with my nerve retractor. I got under the nerve's fine, membranous covering, and slipped both membrane and nerve root gently off the impinging disk. Anticipating my progress, the nurse popped the pituitary rongeur into my right hand—"pituitary" because neurosurgeons use the instrument to excise the diseased pituitary gland, "rongeur" because the instrument bites, which is what the word means in French. Looking something like a scissors with a bent handle, the pituitary rongeur is designed to get down into tight spaces and grasp small structures with its little fishlike mouth. But that little fish mouth has the bite of a shark.

Working the rongeur, I grabbed onto the bulging disk material and tugged at it slightly to see how recalcitrant it might be. Often the protrusion will have all but separated itself from the rest of the disk, which makes things easier. Other times you have to work to get it out. This time it was easy. The culpable material came right out. I got that out of there, then cleaned out a little more to try to preclude any problems down the road. When I was finished, the nerve root plopped right back where it was supposed to be. That always gave me a little jolt of satisfaction, a kind of signal that things were now back in their proper places and all was right with the world. I was certain I had eliminated my patient's leg pain; when she woke up she was going to be all smiles.

I had wondered beforehand how I was going to feel when I walked out of the operating room for the last time. For some of my older friends, bringing their careers to an end had been a sad, even traumatic affair. One of them had had dreams about doing operations for months, dreams that had turned into nightmares. I didn't know if I was going to face anything similar, but as I left the OR I felt great; the timing seemed perfect. And I knew part of that was because I was so looking forward to what was waiting for me next: the students, the medical school's committees, the prospect of doing something about disparate care.

The book *Unequal Treatment* was about ethnic and racial disparities. Strangely, it did not address women's health care and how that compared to the norms. All the more strange because it was well known by then that women, like African Americans and other minority groups, received inferior health care in several important areas.

ONE OF THOSE AREAS was heart disease. In 1999 a group of researchers led by Kevin Schulman, then at Georgetown University Medical School, conducted a large study of cardiac treatment. Schulman's study design was imaginative. Instead of retrospectively subjecting hospital records of cardiac treatment to statistical analysis, Schulman and his colleagues showed a large number of doctors video clips of black, white, male, and female "patients," who were actually actors. All the actors were dressed in hospital gowns, they all gave the same descriptions of their chest pains, and each interview was accompanied by carefully crafted fictitious stress test results.[1]

Schulman's study found that the race and sex of patients influenced physicians' decisions about whether to refer patients for catheterization. Catheterization—the insertion of a thin plastic tube into the arteries and chambers of the heart itself—is the technology that offers the best diagnostic view of coronary disease and is the surest way to tell whether angioplasty or bypass surgery is necessary. If you were black, the report concluded, you were less likely to be referred for catheterization. If you were a woman, you were also less likely to be referred. And if you were a black woman, you were especially less likely to be referred. Given the standardized information the physicians were provided about the patients, the results were striking. The Schulman researchers couldn't do more than speculate about the reasons for these discrepancies. Most probably, they concluded, subconscious bias was at work.

The Schulman study was criticized because, even though the methods and results were clearly presented, the publicity that surrounded its publication exaggerated the disparities. Nevertheless, it became a focal point of discussion about inequalities in cardiac care and helped stimulate the congressional alarm that resulted in *Unequal Treatment*. Although the Institute of Medicine (IOM) book did not look specifically at comparison studies of men and women, it did report black/white comparison studies that included women, and those results reflected the validity of Schulman's conclusions.

Dr. Claudia Thomas, for one, was never skeptical about unequal cardiac care either for women or for African Americans. Thomas is both a woman and an African American. She's also an orthopedic surgeon who currently practices in Florida but who was previously a professor at Johns Hopkins, where she attended medical school. I got to know her when she was an intern and orthopedic resident at Yale during the time I was teaching there.

As a trainee, Claudia stood out in quite a few ways. She was one of the first female orthopedic surgery residents in the country. She was, I think, the very first African American female orthopedic resident, certainly the first ever at Yale (she, like Carlton West and me, was a Wayne Southwick protégé), and she subsequently became the first African American female board-certified orthopedic surgeon. Claudia was also one of those rare individuals who had—and has—no qualms about speaking her mind to those in power. As a Yale intern she became famous for standing up to a cursing, abusive senior surgeon, an absolutely stunning, unheard-of act of brazen rebellion. She apparently told him he should be more civil.[2]

Here's Claudia on what she saw regarding cardiac care while she was training.

"I was a resident, suffering through my two years of general surgery, which were a prerequisite to training in orthopedics. This was at Yale–New Haven Hospital around 1976. Cardiac bypass surgery was in its infancy. It wasn't nearly as common as it is now. The procedure of borrowing veins from the legs, doing the roto-rooter [angioplasty] procedure, rerouting blood supply to the heart—this was relatively new. But it was being done on a regular basis at Yale.

"After my two months of rotating through cardiothoracic surgery, I approached the chairman of the cardiothoracic department and asked him why it was that everyone who was afforded this operation was a white male. New Haven was ethnically diverse, with a significant number of African Americans and a significant number of Hispanics, and, of course, a significant number of women. His mouth dropped open and he looked at me dumbfounded, as if he hadn't even noticed.

"He didn't give me any kind of response. I asked him, 'Is it the case that women don't get this disease?' I wasn't being facetious, because women hadn't been well studied, and I did not know. 'Don't blacks, Hispanics, and women get heart disease? Or do we not?' And he couldn't answer.

"Now, that may possibly have been unconscious bias. But I still think there's a lot of gender bias and a lot of 'fraternal' affinity for your patients if you are a male physician. And a lot of patronizing for your female patients."[3]

That was in the mid-1970s. Here we are, thirty-plus years later and women still receive less of what doctors call "reperfusion," that is, less angioplasty and less bypass surgery. They also, interestingly, receive less in the way of aspirin, beta-blockers, and cholesterol-lowering drugs after they have had a heart attack.[4] Researchers have even found that it can take significantly longer for emergency medical personnel to get women with heart attacks to the hospital.[5]

Some of the reasons for these findings are mysterious.[6] But the consequences can be fatal. Disparities in catheterization and reperfusion, for example, mean that women with heart attacks due to severe blockage of blood flow are almost twice as likely as men to die after a heart attack.[7]

Schulman suggested that subconscious bias was a likely culprit. But women are the mothers, wives, and daughters of mainstream doctors. So where might that come from? It is easy enough to trace the effects of race prejudice and bigotry in medical care. But women, too, suffer from a history of subordination, relegation, and powerlessness, which at the very least suggests that some kind of systemic bias is still at work with this "minority" as well. But is it possible to tease out some of the specifics of how gender bias actually works?

One suggestive study compared physicians' responses to men and women whose reports of their heart symptoms included a mention of stress in their lives. Doctors were more likely to believe that the heart problems of women who reported stress were due to psychological causes, whereas men who talked about stress were considered more likely to have organic heart disease.[8] Psychiatrists tell us that anxiety disorders are more common in women than men. And, of course, women have historically been considered the more emotional sex, less intellectual, less rational—far more likely than men to be driven by feelings rather than by facts. Are these stereotyping factors in play when doctors undertake to diagnose heart disease? Additionally, we know that women of childbearing age are protected to a degree against heart attack by their hormones. Does that too create a mental climate that contributes to less aggressive cardiac care for women generally, older as well as younger?

Something similar may be behind the fact that older women are less likely than men with the same level of kidney disease to receive a transplant. A Johns Hopkins research group conducted a nationwide study of over half a million individuals who developed end-stage renal disease between 2000 and 2005. They found that access to kidney transplants was equal for men and women up to age forty-five. After that, women's access to transplants declined sharply vis-à-vis men, even though women had the same or even higher survival rates after a transplant and so should have been regarded as at least equally qualified candidates. The Hopkins researchers also found that the disparity worsened for women who had other serious health problems along with kidney failure as compared with men who suffered from those same conditions. The lead researcher, Dr. Dorry Segev, a transplant surgeon and the director of clinical research for Hopkins' transplant division, said he believes that nephrologists have a "perceived frailty" about women, which may be shared by women themselves—even though this perception has no basis in fact.[9]

As we know, stereotypes work in various ways. Stereotyping fixes on certain features associated with groups and applies those features to all members of the group. Age-old popular wisdom has it that women are the weaker sex. "Frailty," says Hamlet about his mother, "thy name is woman." Hamlet is talking here about weakness of character. But the phrase resonates on a physical level too. Dr. Segev does not say this directly, but an implication of his study is that there may be an ingrained cultural belief in women's fragility that influences physicians when it comes to considering them as candidates for transplants.

Could that also have something to do with the fact that when women and men have the same level of moderate knee osteoarthritis and pain, women receive fewer joint replacements? Knee osteoarthritis, even before it reaches a critical stage, can be both debilitating and chronically painful. And very often the pain and dysfunction become progressively more severe. In these cases joint replacement is a well-proven, effective treatment that restores mobility and diminishes or eliminates pain. There have been various studies showing that women receive fewer knee replacements than men—a serious disparity. But a breakthrough Canadian study in 2008 focused attention for the first time on why this happens.[10]

The design of the Canadian study resembled that of the Schulman cardiovascular treatment study that was so suggestive about doctors' unconscious prejudices. But instead of using actors in videotaped presentations, the Canadian study used real patients going to see doctors in their offices. Two patients, a man and a woman suffering precisely the same level of knee osteoarthritis, were trained to give doctors identical reports about their pain and disability. They then separately went to see seventy-one family practitioners and orthopedic surgeons. The physicians had volunteered to be included in the study, but were not informed of its purpose and did not know that these particular patients were involved in it. The patients were likewise unaware of the purpose of the study.

In surveys, physicians say that they do not discriminate on the basis of sex. But the results of this study told a different story. For these two individuals, for all practical purposes identical in every way except gender, 67 percent of the physicians who examined them recommended knee replacement for the male patient while only 33 percent did for the female patient.

Commenting on the Canadian study, Dr. Mary O'Connor, orthopedic chair at the Mayo Clinic in Jacksonville, Florida, said, "I think this is not conscious bias. I don't believe those physicians had the female patient in their office and thought, I'm going to withhold a recommendation for surgery. But there's still something going on . . . Do we have a culture that says suffering is permitted in those members of society on whom we place less value? It's okay for women to suffer; they're supposed to suffer? It's okay for poor people and black people to suffer because they're supposed to suffer?"[11]

O'Connor is a leading specialist in joint replacement and bone tumor treatment. She has also been a groundbreaker in the still overwhelmingly male orthopedic community, the first woman member of various orthopedic societies, past president of the Ruth Jackson Society for women orthopedic surgeons, and chair of the Orthopedic Academy's women's health issues committee. As good a surgeon as she is, Mary O'Connor is just as outspoken and blunt on the subject of health-care inequalities.

Disparate care for women is a reality in some areas of orthopedics; at this point many studies have established that indisputably. But O'Connor says we are far from being clear on all the reasons for it. It is not all attributable to bias, either explicit or implicit. In her practice she sees that some women are hesitant about choosing to undergo elective surgeries (as opposed, for instance, to life-saving bone cancer operations). "They will [delay] when they don't feel it's the right time for them to be able to recover. Or if their spouse is ill and they're the primary caregiver, they'll put off surgery." Some researchers have pointed a finger at the different ways men and women tell doctors about their illnesses. "Maybe something [does have] to do with the language of the physician," says O'Connor. "Male patients speak more the language of the physician than female patients. So maybe that lack of common communication makes male patients more comfortable saying, Yes, sign me up for a knee replacement." "We don't have a good understanding of this communication gap," she says. "People come up with all kinds of reasons," but "I don't think there are good studies out there."

Nevertheless, as the Canadian study showed, some sort of physician bias is most definitely at work. Everyone has biases, O'Connor says, as she does herself. "I believe that whatever biases the people had who trained me, I've probably picked up a lot of them." Claudia Thomas makes the same point. "I think we're all biased. You can even be biased against your own race. We all have that cross to bear in our own ways."

Both of these physicians insist that the starting point for dealing with bias is self-awareness. This was Dan Goodenough's conclusion as well. Once doctors recognize that there are both conscious and subconscious forces at work in their relationships with patients, they can take steps to mitigate them. "We have to be vigilant to keep it from affecting the way we practice medicine," says Thomas.

But O'Connor finds that getting that point across to the mostly male orthopedic profession isn't easy. In addition to the educational platform she has made for herself in the Orthopedic Academy, she writes a newsletter column with the tongue-in-cheek title "Putting Sex in Your Orthopedic Practice" (an attempt to increase her readership, she says). Pointing out to her mostly male colleagues that they should be aware they may have an unconscious bias against women may not be, she recognizes, an effective educational strategy. So she takes a roundabout route.

"Let's talk about obese people," she says. "No orthopedic surgeon I know wants to operate on obese people. They're physically harder to operate on. It takes longer. It's more taxing to do the surgery. The risks of complications are higher. They may not want to get up and do their therapies. There's a whole list.

"It's easier to point out that bias. I can say, You know what? I have a bias: I don't like to operate on obese people. I have become conscious that I have that bias. And it's important for me to know that so that I can take action to try to mitigate that bias. We owe it to this patient to try to do our best."

The same is true for women. "There's the stereotypic—Oh, she's going to be a whiner (it's rare that we would ever say that about a male patient). She's going to have a low pain threshold. She's just going to take more of my time and attention to get her through this." Accepting that one bias is at work makes it easier to understand that others may be as well. "I think one of the main messages is that we really need a way to be more sensitive to our internal biases, and trying to make sure that we're not compromising the care of our patients because of those biases."

Claudia Thomas emphasizes the same point. "The most difficult thing to realize is that, yes, *you* may be the one doing it. *You* may be the one guilty of giving different care to people who don't resemble you . . . There's a lot of bias and sexism that exist within everybody. It's hard to have that breakthrough where people realize that it *is* them." I'd add that it's especially hard to believe given that our mothers, wives, and daughters are women. Yet it's no less true for that.

Older women have less access to transplants than their male age-mates. But older people in general are often subjected to different treatment than their younger fellows. Among the various groups that experience disparate care, the elderly are conspicuous.

For women and for African Americans, biased treatment is often due to implicit stereotypes and prejudices. Many studies have demonstrated that the elderly are also subject to bias and stereotyping, but the reasons they receive different care are by and large far more obvious and self-evident. Older people are often burdened by several illnesses at the same time. They may communicate poorly or be less aware; they may be suffering some level of dementia. They may be reliant on family members to serve as intermediaries with doctors. All these elements make them more difficult to treat—"medically complex absorbers of time and resources," as one practitioner put it. Emergency room personnel may have a tendency to pigeonhole them as "train wrecks" or "disasters waiting to happen," seeing the elderly in terms of the excessive burdens they impose on those who care for them.[12]

Dr. Jack Rowe is one of America's leading experts on medicine and aging. Now a professor at the Columbia University School of Public Health, he was formerly CEO of Mt. Sinai in New York and then of the Aetna Insurance Company. He recalls that he got interested in geriatrics while he was still in training. "I realized," he says, "that the elderly were just not receiving the degree of attention and the sophisticated approach to health care that was warranted . . . they weren't being treated with the dignity they deserved."

Rowe saw the same attitudes on general hospital rounds that were evident in the emergency room. "In many ways," he says, "it was considered that the resources expended on the elderly were wasted."[13]

Some researchers have studied the ageist attitudes of health-care providers and their effects on outcomes. Others, like Yale psychologist Becca Levy, have found that implicit ageism is internalized by the elderly themselves as well as by their juniors, and that when negative stereotypes are directed inward they can have startlingly negative consequences. Older individuals, she says, who have positive self-perceptions of aging live seven and a half years longer than those with negative images. If she is correct, it means that internalized perceptions are more significant than blood pressure, cholesterol level, smoking, exercise, and body mass in terms of extending life.[14] The power of the mind, that supposedly unquantifiable catalyst that so many practitioners, myself included, have endeavored to mobilize in our treatment, is perhaps not so unquantifiable after all.

Levy notes that there are differences between the internalized stereotyping of the elderly and of blacks and women, in particular that the elderly have fewer available defense mechanisms. But she believes that there is a fundamental commonality as well. "To the extent," she says, "that the process is shared, there is a greater likelihood that the outcome will be as well."[15] Frantz Fanon so many years ago described the colonialized mentality as a phenomenon that affects the psyche of devalued people. Since then a significant literature has developed on racism as an underlying cause of disease. And here, with the aged, we can begin to see the stark physiological impact of self-perception as well.

Jack Rowe was drawn to geriatric medicine when he was struck by the lack of normal consideration and respect accorded older patients. But his research background led him to explore the biomedical rather than the psychological dimension of the mistreatment he was seeing.

Rowe had spent two years at NIH studying the physiological effects of aging on various organ systems and metabolic processes. So when he came back to his residency at Boston's Beth Israel Hospital, he brought a different awareness to the problems of ageism. "I did not come to geriatric medicine," he says, "from the point of view of someone who was just sympathetic to the dignity part of it or to the human rights part of it, the fairness part. I came to it from a science base. No one had studied the elderly. They were often given the wrong doses of medicine, for example, simply because people did not understand. I said, this needs to be studied. The information that's developed has to be incorporated into the practice of medicine so that the proper care can be given. Just like in pediatrics, you don't just say children *deserve* attention. No, children need to be studied so that we *know* what the proper dose is." "We have pediatrics," he told the chairman of his department. "We need geriatrics. Old people are not just old adults any more than children are young adults; they're different."

That was in 1978, at just about the same time I arrived at Beth Israel's orthopedic service. In response to Rowe's arguments, Beth Israel gave him the resources to establish a program in aging. After that, Harvard Medical School tapped him to organize a division on aging that introduced geriatric education into the curriculum for the first time and developed into a large program of research and clinical training.

One result was the beginning of a paradigm shift in the treatment of older people's health problems. It was then, and still is, all too common to consider many morbidities affecting the elderly as merely a matter of getting old rather than as disease entities that should be addressed just as they would be addressed in a younger person. The story gerontologists tell to illustrate this is about the elderly man who tells his doctor that his knee hurts. The doctor says, "It's just old age." "Funny," says the man, "my other knee's also eighty-two, and it doesn't hurt at all." Many conditions, says Rowe, "that are attributed to 'old age' in fact are disease, which needs to be understood in the presence of an older person's body." As much as anything, ageism in medical care is perpetuated by the relegation of the elderly into a category where the possibility of treatment seems just not so compelling as it is for others.

The bottom line for scientists such as Becca Levy and Jack Rowe, whether or not they state it explicitly, is about the value of life itself, which old age throws into high relief in a way almost nothing else can. Should the elderly and their health providers consider older lives to be somehow of less value because elders have already had a decently long run and because the end is, in any event, relatively close by?

That is, in fact, the major debate that has both divided and puzzled the health-care world for several decades already and is quickly growing sharper than ever. In 1987 bioethicist Daniel Callahan wrote a book entitled *Setting Limits: Medical Goals in an Aging Society.* He argued there that burgeoning costs for medical care constituted a looming financial crisis for the country. Given that, some kind of health-care rationing was necessary. Limits had to be set, and the best way to do that would be by using age as a cutoff point— somewhere around eighty was his original suggestion. Older people consume a large share of the available resources, especially for expensive procedures such as cardiac surgery, dialysis, and transplants. And often these provide only a brief elongation of frail and sickly lives. "Something or other is going to get us in the long run," he said in a later interview, arguing that people should simply accept that rather than succumb "to the lure of a slightly longer life."[16]

Jack Rowe is one of many experts on aging who take a different view. "Age is a convenient marker," he says, "because it is a proxy for function. Ninety-year-olds are less likely to contribute to society than forty-year-olds, more likely to be impaired, etc, etc. The problem for individuals who would like to use age as a criterion is the tremendous variability with advancing age in functional status. You can find seventy- and seventy-five-year-olds who function as well as the average thirty-year-old. That is the moral hazard associated with an age-based criterion. It doesn't take into account the functional capacity of the individual and doesn't recognize that the functional capacity varies dramatically with advancing age."

Neither of these arguments addresses such issues as the extent to which society should feel obligated to provide maximum care for its elderly because of their past contributions, including nurturing and educating younger generations. But whether age or functionality is the criterion for cutting off expensive treatments, both arguments do ask us to assess the value of individual life against the apparent good of the larger society seen in terms of the dedication of health resources to its younger, more productive members. The fact that this is such a thorny moral dilemma explains why the question of rationing is still so hotly debated, even as health costs continue to spiral. "Is it the same thing to die old as to die young?" asks the protagonist of Euripides' play *Alcestis*. He has just asked his aged father to take his place in death, and his father has refused to do it. "Yes," the father says. "We have only one life to live and not two." "You like the sunlight. Don't you think your father does? I count the time I have to spend in death as long, and the time I have left to live as little. But that little is sweet."

The moral issue posed by the problem of rationing health care perplexes moral philosophers, let alone doctors and policy makers. But it does focus attention like a laser on the great underlying question: What does it mean to value life? Is everyone's life equally worthwhile? What, if anything, can justify devaluing the lives of the old, sickly, and nonproductive relative to the lives of those who are younger, fitter, and more productive? And if the elderly, then what about the severely disabled, another group that suffers inequities in health care, or even those somewhat less severely disabled?

It's one thing to look at questions like these as problems at the intersection of morality and public health policy that will, if thinkers like Daniel Callahan are right, require careful decision making. But the existing disparities in health care tell us that our society has been making decisions right along that some groups' lives are less valuable than others—without anything at all in the way of careful or even conscious decision making.

WHEN WE LOOK AT RACE AND GENDER, we see that powerful implicit biases are at work, conditioned in over extremely long periods. Moving toward equality for African Americans and women means, first of all, becoming aware, expanding our understanding of who we are and how our minds work. Other groups suffering from disparities reveal different barriers that test our ability to treat each other as equals, that is, to recognize the equal value of life. Latinos are one such group. Gays and lesbians are another.

Hispanic Americans receive inferior care in a number of significant areas. They get less in the way of angioplasty and bypass surgery and they have less access to mental health care.[17] They don't receive basic recommended health-care services for which they are eligible at the same rate as majority whites, including mammograms, Pap smears, colonoscopies, cardiovascular screening, flu vaccines, and diabetes screening.[18]

The study showing that blacks receive less pain medication for long bone fractures was secondary to an earlier study comparing Hispanics and non-Hispanic whites—that showed similar disparities.

It seems clear from the fracture study and other studies on the disparate use of medication in cancer pain and in childbearing that built-in biases are operating. "[These] lead me to suspect," says Massachusetts General Hospital professor and senior scientist at the Institute for Health Policy Joseph Betancourt, "that there are certain assumptions being made about those patients . . . Clinicians want to believe and are trained to believe that we don't treat patients differently and that we don't stereotype. But there's a significant culture in medicine that does stereotype people based on any variety of characteristics, whether it be insurance, socioeconomic status, physical size, race, ethnicity, or sexual orientation. There's almost this built-in 'good patient/bad patient,' the bad patient being one where you have to take extra steps to sort things out. I think that's just the way the medical system is set up. That's the deeply ingrained culture that we see."[19]

But Betancourt, who is of Puerto Rican origin, explains that the culture of the patient plays its role in the equation as well. "Culturally—not to make any generalizations; I think this is an issue that crosses cultures—certain patients may have different styles of communication that might impede effective communication and care. I've had many patients who, because I'm the doctor, have not wanted to bother me when they've had chest pains or shortness of breath. Their view of the doctor is someone you don't bother. If you have a problem, you just go to the emergency room. I've had patients whom I have explained things to, and they say, Yes, doctor, yes doctor all the way through. Then, when I've checked to make sure they understood, they really haven't. That's because of their view of the physician as a respected figure."[20]

The factors behind disparate care are complex and often difficult to sort out. The Hispanic community itself is made up of numerous nationalities whose cultures can differ in important ways, which magnifies the complexity. But all speak Spanish, and many have a limited, or sometimes nonexistent, command of English.

The large study I mentioned above by Eric Cheng and his colleagues on the receipt of preventive health care showed that Hispanic patients who spoke English at home received care at almost the same level as white non-Hispanic patients. Hispanic patients who were comfortable in English but spoke Spanish at home were significantly less likely to receive the same care, and patients who did not speak English at home and were not comfortable speaking English were far less likely to receive equal care.

Language, says Betancourt, along with every doctor who treats Hispanic patients, plays an essential role. Language not only enables communication, language is a marker for acculturation. When non-Hispanic doctors (that is, the vast majority) treat Spanish-speaking patients with limited English, they find themselves in an alien space, disabled from communicating effectively and as unfamiliar with the patient's cultural norms and expectations as the patient might be with the doctor's.

Leonor Fernandez is an internist, another colleague of mine at Harvard. "I think Latinos expect a different style of relating," she says. "They can often find doctors here to be cold and disinterested. Of course, many Latinos have grown up in America. So it depends on what group you are talking to. The biggest divide is whether they're recent immigrants or not, or English speaking or not.

"I see about a sixty percent immigrant population. I think the big issues are comfort and language. If they need an interpreter, it's harder to get a visit because they have to coordinate more people's schedules. It takes longer. There's less privacy because here's another person in the visit. There's a million things. And depending on the quality of the interpreter, a lot of the information can be lost in translation.

"So the one two three reason they come to me is that they'd rather communicate directly in Spanish, or, for those who speak English, they feel more comfortable. I also have several Latinos who speak English to me, but they come because they feel that there's a higher likelihood of allegiance. They say, *'You* know how we are.'"[21]

When doctors are working in stressful environments, under time and cost pressures, when they have inadequate support, when their training has conditioned them to focus on the prescriptive side of medicine—that is when they rely most on stereotyping, the mind's natural cognitive shortcut. And that, says Betancourt, together with the IOM researchers, is how many of the disparities we see get themselves embedded into our national health care. "This is not an indictment of physicians," Betancourt writes, "but instead a call to action and open-mindedness."[22]

Fernandez, with her mixed practice of Hispanics and non-Hispanics, has thought for years about what open-mindedness actually entails. "The more social difference," she says, "the more difficult it is for you to identify with that person sitting there, the more likely you are not to make that extra effort to figure it out." That extra effort, she explains, means having Spanish speakers on staff if you yourself don't speak the language. It means being aware that poor people may not be able to pay for expensive antibiotics, that they may not be able to call back and explain what their problem is, that they may find it harder or impossible to take more time off from work for a return visit that can require a long trip on public transportation. "You [the doctor] have to be able to take account," she says. "You have to have 'anticipatory guidance' on these things—you have to anticipate them and figure out in advance a way of dealing with them."

Joseph Kramer is a pediatrician and family doctor who is a model, as much as anyone I know about, of the doctor who "knows what it means." Retired now, for thirty-five years Joe Kramer was the only private physician on New York's Lower East Side. His patients were almost all Hispanic and black. His office was in a lobby-level two-bedroom apartment in the Jacob Riis housing projects on Avenue D.

Kramer, a non-Spanish-speaker, left a pediatric group in a wealthy New Jersey suburb, which he found less than satisfying, in order to hang out his shingle in a neighborhood that had an abundance of children and little in the way of health care. "When I got there," he says, "I knew a little high school Spanish. I had a dictionary. Then I figured, This is stupid. How can you practice medicine if you can't talk to the patients? So I picked up a good amount of medical Spanish. Then, when I'd get stuck, I'd always call in [receptionists] Sonia or Maria. And I'd listen very carefully to the conversation. To make sure they weren't making up their own questions. 'Just ask them what I want you to ask them.' I learned a lot by listening to the questions and to the answers. I picked up the Spanish."[23]

Kramer became a fixture in the neighborhood. He was an advocate for his patients. He knew not just their medical complaints, but their problems and their lives. He charged them what they could afford. If it was necessary, he'd stop everything to rush a kid over to the Bellevue Hospital emergency room. He could sympathize with his patients or yell at them if he thought they needed it. He knew how to talk to them. NYU, Columbia Presbyterian, and Cornell rotated medical students through his office so they could see what "real" doctoring was like. "As far as I'm concerned," Kramer says, "it's all a matter of respect for your fellow human being. People are poor. They're looked upon as being the pariahs of society because they're poor, because they have strange-sounding last names or a different skin color. They're always looked down on. I don't know what's such a big deal about treating a human being like a human being."[24]

Not all doctors are going to be Joseph Kramers, but his attitude should give each of us reason to pause for a moment and think about how we conduct our practices. "You have to be able to talk about things and listen empathetically," says Leonor Fernandez, and Kramer was able to both talk and listen, which went far toward making him the exceptional physician he was.

PROVIDING EQUAL TREATMENT for patients from non-English-speaking communities requires an accommodating mind-set and the ability to regard "extra effort" not as something outside the norm, but as a necessary part of a doctor's practice. "Extra effort" is the sine qua non in all human relationships where different people and groups come to each other within a civil society that values equality. But it is most especially a requirement in the special relationship between doctors and patients, where doctors have taken on themselves the obligation to heal.

In treating Hispanics, equality-conscious physicians must enlarge their horizons to accommodate language and culture. In treating sexual minority patients, equality conscious physicians have to stretch themselves in other ways that their training and conditioning have not necessarily prepared them for.

The CDC document *Healthy People 2010* identifies gay, lesbian, bisexual, and transgendered (GLBT) people as a group that experiences disparate health care. The communities we have discussed already—blacks, women, the elderly, and Hispanics—are all clearly identifiable by physical markers or, in the case of Hispanics, by language use and family names. But sexual minorities are not necessarily identifiable at all. And if doctors are not aware of their patients' sexual orientation, they will simply not provide appropriate health care. Disparate care for sexual minority patients is not a matter of unequal treatment for the same diseases and conditions. It is a matter of not receiving the same level of appropriate care that mainstream patients receive. Sexual minorities are subject to deep and sometimes violent cultural biases that have severe consequences in terms of elevated suicide levels among adolescents and higher rates of smoking and alcoholism among adults. But "the real issue," says the Fenway Institute's Harvey Makadon, "is what do people feel comfortable telling doctors, and how do you get that information. It's not a traditional disparity . . . It's an invisibility."[25]

Makadon is one of the country's leading voices on the health care of sexual minorities. An internist at Beth Israel and professor of medicine at Harvard, he came out to his own doctor at age forty. "I was disappointed by the lack of discussion following my emotionally difficult statement about my sexual orientation," Makadon recalls. "He did not discuss my sexual history or recommend that I be tested for HIV, nor did we discuss the need for hepatitis A or B immunizations."[26] Makadon's experience wasn't unique. Having treated many sexual minority individuals in his clinical work, he found that most had never had frank discussions with their doctors before.

While it's not possible to guess numbers for GLBT individuals whose medical encounters do not include an exploration of sexual behavior, we do have some fix on the number of gay, lesbian, and bisexual persons in the country. The 2005 American Community Survey of the U.S. Census Bureau found that 8.8 million adults self-identify as either gay, lesbian, or bisexual. While homosexual women have several health issues relating to their sexuality (mental health problems, possible inadequacy of Pap smear screening, and potentially higher risk for breast cancer, for example), male homosexuals are at special risk from a variety of ailments that are rarely noticed in primary care examinations where sexual orientation has remained a closed topic. CDC health-care guidelines call for routine screening for HIV and other viral and bacterial STDs including syphilis, gonorrhea, and chlamydia, and for hepatitis A and B vaccination. Human papilloma viruses are also transmitted sexually and are common in male homosexuals. Human papilloma viruses cause genital and anal warts. But it is not nearly as well known, even among physicians, that the strains of HPV implicated in cervical cancer can also cause anal carcinomas, which are being seen more and more often.[27]

Unless doctors are aware of their patients' sexual orientation, such illnesses may not be discovered until they reach advanced stages. Yet, fearful of censure and discrimination, gays, lesbians, and bisexuals often keep these identifications very private. That tendency is even more marked among some minority groups that are especially intolerant of homosexuality. Among African Americans, for example, there is an underground syndrome known as the "down low." Men on the down low identify as heterosexual and typically have wives or girlfriends but at the same time carry on secret sexual relationships with other men. The HIV-AIDS epidemic is particularly prevalent in the African American community, with troubling numbers of infections among black women. Researchers speculate that the spike in women's rates may well be related to men with this concealed bisexual orientation.[28]

The challenge, of course, is for physicians to find ways to bring the subject of sexuality into the normal course of clinical interaction. Routine interviews in primary care medicine rarely more than touch on a patient's sexual history. The issues of sexual identity and practices are unlikely to come up, not just because patients may be reticent, but because doctors themselves find it awkward and difficult to ask those kinds of questions. We tend to stay away from subjects that make us uncomfortable, and in this doctors aren't different from the rest of us. Their responsibility to care for their patients, though, has consequences that do set them apart, in this area as in others.

Makadon emphasizes this issue in the papers he writes and talks he gives. "You have to understand," he tells doctors, "that you cannot just make assumptions. You have to ask basic questions. And the most important thing is that you have to feel comfortable that you can ask personal questions, as long as you are respectful of individuals and you are empathic and nonjudgmental."

At Harvard Medical School, Makadon teaches the first-year course in medical interviewing. The traditional approach has been to leave the social and family dimension to the end, but he is changing the format. "We start off the history," he explains, "with what we refer to as a mini-social history. We call it Getting to Know the Patient as a Person. You should consider," he tells students, "if the best way to begin isn't 'What brings you here today,' but 'Why don't we start off by telling me a little bit about yourself so I can get to know something about you and your life.' A lot of people, given that open opportunity to talk about themselves, are much more likely to talk about the fact that 'Well, I'm in a relationship.' "

"Most of all," he says, "you can actually be curious about people's lives and ask them questions. And usually you're going to be fine with that. But it does require a certain mind-set. That you are willing and comfortable at talking to people."

Reluctance to discuss sexual identity and practice is a barrier to equal health care for sexual minorities. Achieving ease in these matters can be a stretch for physicians. But in the end it is, perhaps, no more of a stretch than other kinds of mind-opening and practice-altering processes that are fundamental if we are to make significant progress toward equal treatment. In the last analysis, if you value one patient as much as another, that's an effort you simply have to make.

AS I CLOSED DOWN my surgical career, these were the kinds of issues and themes I knew were going to absorb my attention into the future. My overriding thought in terms of how to start dealing with them was that the subject of disparities in health care should somehow be brought into the medical school curriculum. With that in mind I went to Dean Lowenstein to suggest that we set up a committee to explore what might be possible. "That sounds like a reasonable idea," he said. "Why don't you get a couple of people together to look into it?"

12

CULTURALLY COMPETENT CARE

I will keep the sick from harm and injustice.

—From the Hippocratic Oath

ONCE I HAD THE BLESSING of Dean Lowenstein, I forged ahead with the committee project. Almost immediately Dan Goodenough agreed to take part, as did Roxana Llerena-Quinn, a psychologist who had partnered with Dan in creating their course on self-awareness. Then others came forward. Before I knew it, I had gathered a core group of ten faculty and key administrators.

As word got around that a committee on health disparities was forming, more people began knocking on my door. It was almost as if the medical school had just been waiting for something like this. Clinicians and medical scientists were reading an ever-growing number of disturbing studies on the subject, and many of them obviously wanted to do something about it. Given the response, it seemed all they needed was an entity to relate to and some leadership. Within a short period we had fifty-plus committee members, which soon grew to ninety. I had more talent and enthusiasm on board than I could have hoped for.

As master of the Holmes Society I was also ex officio on the medical school's other committees, so in a sense I had a whole institution to work with. Besides that, the medical school had just then instituted a wide-ranging "blue skies" review of the entire curriculum. Everything was open for discussion: courses, teaching techniques, philosophies of medical education. The school was in ferment, like nothing I had seen before—opening itself up to new, out-of-the-mainstream ideas. It was as if circumstances were conspiring in my favor. I could practically feel the wind at my back.

With the scope of the racial, ethnic, gender, and other biases and their destructive consequences revealing themselves more or more clearly, I was also feeling a sense of urgency. To me and the others in our core group, this was not some kind of diffuse, intractable problem that we could only hope might improve over time. We knew then—in 2001 and 2002—as we still know today, that even while we were talking, African Americans in emergency rooms were not receiving adequate analgesics, women brought into hospitals with heart attacks were dying because of disparities in treatment, Spanish-speaking Americans were struggling to figure out when and how they should take their diabetes medications. Sitting there at the medical school, there might be little we could do right off in terms of national health-care policy—but Harvard being Harvard, we could at least try to take the lead on some meaningful strategies that would bring equal care into the training and thought processes of medical students and faculty.

There were strong signs that momentum was growing nationally for exactly those goals. Just as we were gathering momentum, the Liaison Committee on Medical Education (the national accreditation agency for American and Canadian medical schools) issued two new directives. Directive 21 stipulated:

> Faculty and students must demonstrate an understanding of the manner in which people of diverse cultures and belief systems perceive health and illness and respond to various symptoms, diseases, and treatments.

Directive 22 read:

> Medical students must learn to recognize and appropriately address gender and cultural biases in themselves and others, and in the process of health care delivery.

Notably, the directives read "must" rather than "should"—"faculty and students must . . . ," the Liaison Committee's way of emphasizing that these were not suggestions but hard requirements.

The directives addressed two principal problems: physician and trainee lack of understanding and sensitivity toward groups outside the mainstream, and medical students' need to become aware of their own biases and how they bear on health care. I hadn't had anything to do with these Liaison Committee formulations, but they reflected the same conclusions I and others engaged with these issues had arrived at ourselves. There was, clearly, a groundswell going on in the medical establishment. The only question was how best to make ourselves part of it.

We had momentum. What we didn't have was money. Dean Lowenstein had given me his approval but hadn't provided any resources to go along with it, which was a recipe for a lot of talk and no action. If we were going to get anything concrete accomplished, it seemed pretty clear I was going to have to find the funding for it myself.

Joan Reede, the medical school's dean of diversity, saw her way to getting us part of a grant. Then John Ruffin, director of NIH's Center for Minority Health and Health Disparities, figured out a way to fast-track some moderate support. The Gladden Society came through with a contribution, and I managed to muster a few other donations. But that still left us well short of what I thought we needed.

Wondering where I might raise additional funds, I found myself talking with Sam Thier, president of Partners—the health-care system anchored by Massachusetts General and Brigham and Women's Hospitals. "Why don't I introduce you to Cleve Killingsworth?" Sam said. "He's just come to town as president of Blue Cross Blue Shield. You should meet him, if only to welcome him. He's African American; I'm sure he'd appreciate the gesture."

Feeling like an old Boston hand, I arranged to see Cleve Killingsworth, to welcome him to the city and to the city's black community. We chatted about our backgrounds, his in the health-care industry, mine in medicine. I told him how I was now retired from surgery and how excited I was about our new committee. I mentioned what I was hoping to do, some of the people I had with me, and how I was still in the fund-raising stage. I wasn't planning to ask Killingsworth for money; this was just a welcoming meeting, brother to brother. But as I was about to leave, he said, "By the way, would fifty thousand dollars help?"

To people experienced with fund-raising this might sound completely ordinary. A person with money in his budget hears about a project he likes, and even though he isn't being directly solicited, decides to make a contribution. In the world of philanthropy it probably happens twenty times a day. That is, it probably happens twenty times a day in the white world. In the black world, or at least in my world, Cleve's offer was astonishing. It wasn't the money itself; I was so emotionally taken I almost forgot about the number. It was the fact that here I was, standing in the office of the black president of a huge corporation, and this African American man had the power to just spontaneously make a gesture like this. That seemed to me momentous, something I could never have imagined. This was the opposite of the colonialized mentality that I saw only too often in blacks' relations with other blacks. We are now, as I'm writing this, seven years further down the line, so it's possible things have changed a bit, or maybe more than a bit. But back then it just blew me away.

With Cleve's donation, the committee was really up and running. I had decided that we should call ourselves the Culturally Competent Care Committee. The idea of culturally competent medical care had been around since at least the late 1970s. In practice, as opposed to theory, the concept began with efforts to deal with the cultural and linguistic challenges of providing health care to non-English-speaking immigrants.[1] Early on, it gained traction in some nursing schools and local community health centers. But I believe the obstetrician-gynecologists were the first physicians to take it seriously, which stands to reason since at that time they were a mostly male group caring for women, so they needed to understand something about a psychological universe different from their own.

I myself had picked up the idea of competence—though not cultural competence—from Steve Smith, who had been a highly innovative dean of medical education at Brown University. Smith had injected a new way of thinking into the Brown medical school curriculum (which I was advising on as a member of the school's visiting committee). Traditionally, medical school curricula are grounded on the basic medical sciences in the first years and on so-called clerkships in the later years. These third- and fourth-year clerkships give students clinical experiences in medicine, surgery, pediatrics, obstetrics, and other specialties. Steve's approach was to focus on the competencies that would be required of a doctor in practice rather than just on the different medical disciplines. A trained physician needed to be competent in taking histories, doing physical exams, interpreting lab work, reading X-rays, making differential diagnoses, and performing in other specific areas. As dean he pushed to reorient the curriculum, and though he wasn't completely successful, the idea of competencies made headway at Brown and began circulating though the medical college world. Steve was and is considered the architect of the competency approach to medical education.

The competency approach began to spread into other areas of medicine too, and at some point people began to talk about cultural competency. The idea was that just as doctors need to know how to take a history and do a physical exam, in order to provide good care they should also have a basic sense of their patients' social and cultural circumstances. Unequal care thrives on differences between doctors and their patients, on poor communication, on stereotyping, on misconnections in the relationship between the two. "The more difference," as Leonor Fernandez says, "the more difficult it is for the doctor to identify with that person sitting there."[2]

Some of Fernandez's Hispanic patients tell her, "You know how we are." African American patients, Alvin Poussaint says, often looked to make a connection with him, black patient to black doctor.

We know that patients of the same race and ethnicity as their doctors tend to trust them more and derive greater satisfaction from their interactions.[3] But given the relatively small number of minority doctors, most minority patients are treated by mainstream, white doctors. Culturally competent care education, we thought, would be one powerful way to help mainstream doctors bridge the gap between themselves and their minority patients. If doctors are culturally literate they will feel more comfortable with these patients, which inevitably elicits more patient comfort with them and consequently greater patient satisfaction.

Physicians should be aware, for example, that many African Americans come to a doctor's office with a degree of distrust, that we might be particularly sensitive to suggestions of disrespect or condescension. Physicians should be aware that Hispanic patients may be especially deferential and may not press to understand everything they should understand. They should know that people from some Asian societies may be more fatalistic about their illnesses than people born and raised in America might be, and that Muslim ideas of propriety can make physical examinations of female patients by male physicians problematic. Knowledge of this sort is not meant to be reductionist—to define individual patients according to their group identities. But no doctor wants to embarrass, insult, or misunderstand his patients out of ignorance. For physicians who have patients from specific minority communities, a basic awareness of cultural tendencies is essential.

More broadly, training in cultural competence stimulates an awareness of the extent to which culture plays a role in a patient's understanding of health care. Cultural competence emphasizes the importance to doctors of listening to their patients with sensitivity to who they are. It focuses attention on a doctor's ability to communicate, which we know correlates not just with comfort and trust, but with adherence to therapeutic regimens and treatment outcomes.[4]

At bottom, cultural awareness helps to validate people who belong to groups other than our own, people who might otherwise be devalued or disregarded, even if subconsciously. Cultural competence allows physicians to understand with greater clarity that individuals in such groups sometimes act and think differently—about medicines, about health, about doctors, about human relations in general. But these differences in perception and understanding are not due to deficiencies of some kind; they are due to the fact that these patients' communities have different histories, environments, and circumstances of life that beg to be understood if doctors are to communicate effectively with them and to provide them with the best care they can.

I was convinced that training medical students and faculty in this area would open minds and, by bettering patient-doctor communication across racial and ethnic lines, would help improve minority care. Some recent research has even indicated that physicians who are good at showing respect for their patients, at informing them effectively, and at supporting their involvement *"can transcend issues of race and sex"* (italics mine).[5] That is to say, though black patients do tend to feel more trust with black doctors, white doctors who are good at cross-cultural communication can more than make up for racial differences. As the authors of one study put it, "communication, more so than racial concordance, [is] related to patients' perceptions of a personal connection with their physicians, as well as to patient outcomes."[6]

Cultural awareness can go a long way toward breaking down barriers on the doctor's side of the medical encounter. But patients, especially minority patients, bring their own communication difficulties into the doctor's office. Differences in socioeconomic status, educational levels, and manner of speaking magnify the divide between patient and doctor and typically lead to less patient engagement, less patient satisfaction, and worse outcomes.[7]

But we know that personal interest, respect, and openness on the doctor's side create a powerful reciprocal effect. And this is true, of course, not just for doctors and patients who face each other over a cultural divide, but for all doctors and patients. Debra Roter and Judith Hall emphasize that "much of what a person does in interaction is in response to a triggering behavior by the other person."[8]

The more comfortable a white doctor feels with a black or Hispanic patient, the easier and more effective her communication is likely to be—and the easier and more effective the patient's own communication will be. No less an authority than the Dalai Lama tells us that approaching others with an expectation that they will be good, kind, friendly, and so on dictates their behavior to some degree. It potentiates their response in the desired direction. The medical encounter is no different.[9]

Our committee's main mission, I thought, would be to find ways to institutionalize culturally competent care. I wanted to integrate cultural awareness into the medical school's educational mainstream. With so many hands available, we split into subcommittees to come up with proposals for faculty training, curriculum reform, outreach and communication within Harvard's vast healthcare establishment and with other institutions, and to develop evaluative tools to measure the effects of culturally competent care. All of this was aimed at overcoming the implicit categorization of minority communities as somehow less worthy and the bias that perception inevitably triggers.

I was buoyed in these efforts by the fact that all our culturally competent care initiatives could be seen as addressing the Liaison Committee's Directive 21—the requirement for medical students and doctors to understand diverse cultures. This directive had grown out of the burgeoning diversity in American life, where minorities composed of African Americans, Latinos, Asian Americans, and others were becoming an ever-greater percentage of the nation's population. Directive 21 meant that students and faculty needed to look outward to sharpen their vision and their understanding of the diverse cultures that increasingly made up the American social fabric and, consequently, doctors' caseloads. Directives 21 and 22 together were going to force Harvard and other medical schools to look positively at just the kinds of programs we were incubating.

The Liaison Committee's Directive 22 was in a sense the obverse of Directive 21. If Directive 21 asked students to look outward, Directive 22 invited them to look inward, to recognize and examine their own cultural and gender biases. This was exactly the subject Roxana Llerena-Quinn and Dan Goodenough had been engaged with for a number of years. The course on self-awareness they had developed anticipated the Liaison Committee's requirement and addressed it directly.

Roxana Llerena-Quinn was a clinical psychologist with many years of experience in community health centers. She had developed mental health programs for Latinos and was working at Children's Hospital when Harvard asked her to come in as part of its response to an incident that had riveted the medical school's attention on racial and ethnic relations.

The incident happened at a school Halloween party. Two white students had come to the party made up as Clarence Thomas and Anita Hill—makeup-darkened faces and all—which an African American student found insulting. The African American student explained why and asked them to leave, then he left himself. When he came back to find the white students still there and still in their costumes, he slugged the white male. In the midst of considerable publicity, the administration ordered suspensions and other disciplinary action. More importantly, the event seemed to crystallize racial tensions that had been brewing beneath the surface.

To help address the underlying problems, the school hired Llerena-Quinn to work with Dan Goodenough and others. A series of focus groups that involved students and faculty resulted in a consensus that multiculturalism should be incorporated into the curriculum—not necessarily as a stand-alone, mandatory course, but rather as an element in at least some established courses or clerkships.

"So there was a consensus," Llerena-Quinn remembers. "But there was also resistance and avoidance. 'This is wonderful,' teaching faculty told us, 'but there's no time in my course. Besides, a broken bone is a broken bone.'"[10]

Llerena-Quinn and her colleagues had run straight into the brick wall of medicine's prescriptive culture, which says, implicitly and explicitly, that biomedical and physiological markers count for everything significant while the psychosocial dimension of a patient's diagnosis and treatment is more or less irrelevant. In this view, a certain amount of lip service to multiculturalism might be in order, but when it comes down to it, concrete action is seen as burdensome and unnecessary.

But the multicultural group were not deterred. They asked themselves why people were so reluctant to engage with such an obvious need. How might they encourage students and faculty to break through the cultural and personal inhibitions that surrounded issues of prejudice and stereotyping? And they began to conceptualize a course. "One idea was to get people more comfortable in talking about differences," Llerena-Quinn says. "But as long as we study others, there's a tendency to stereotype or generalize. We miss the individuality. So let's look at variables as they pertain to ourselves. Let's use ourselves as the object of study."[11] The result was the creation of what I thought was an extraordinary course in self-awareness.

When I first heard about the course I asked if I could sit in. But Roxana and Dan were reluctant. For students and faculty to explore their own biases, they needed an intimate, protective environment, which precluded outside observers. So I asked if I could take the course myself, to which the answer was, "Of course." So at the age of sixty-six I became a student.

The course was a revelation. As we went through the readings, videos, and intimate discussions on racial, ethnic, gender, religious, and other group identity issues, I was more and more impressed with how we students began to grasp the force of culture in shaping our own identities, and how this enabled us to understand better the complexities of others' identities. More knowledge and insight brought a heightened sense of empathy, and in the process we became attuned to what our own biases were and where they came from. And as we became more insightful about fellow students from different backgrounds, races, and groups, our stereotypes began to fall away.

One fundamental element of the course was an exercise called the cultural genogram, which came from Roxana's field of family therapy. Essentially a detailed map of one's own cultural heritage and identity, the genogram is widely used as a training mechanism to help raise cultural awareness and sensitivity among therapists.[12] The process asks students to identify the ethnic, racial, gender, class, religious, sexual orientation, and other influences that constitute their family's and their own understanding of where they come from, who they are, and why they think of others the way they do. Creating a map of this sort is a demanding and revealing process, and when small, intimate groups of students from different heritages share their cultural genograms, complexity and individuality emerge to take the place of generalization and stereotype.

This was, I thought, the very basic science of cultural competence. Just as students have to understand biochemistry and physiology before they can understand disease, culturally competent doctors have to get a sense for their own cultures before they can grasp the meaning of culture for others. And the cultural genogram exercise revealed that understanding even our own cultural identity goes well beyond the pat, automatic knowledge most of us assume we have.

Constructing and sharing genograms can have a dramatic impact on stereotyping. The exercise stimulates the process social psychologists call "mindfulness," which is the disposition to make active distinctions about others. In one famous study, sixth-graders who had been experimentally inculcated with mindfulness became less likely to discriminate against handicapped children and less likely to want to avoid them than a control group was. The mindful children were more inclined to see the handicapped children in terms of their individuality rather than in terms of their disabilities.[13]

In a more recent experiment along these lines, psychologists tested a group of random people recruited at a laundromat in Boston to see if inducing mindfulness could affect stereotypes about the elderly. The subjects were divided into groups. Each group was shown photographs of old and young people. One group was asked to sort the photographs four times, giving each pictured individual four different attributes. For example, a subject might distinguish individuals in the photographs as old or young, intelligent or unintelligent, friendly or aggressive, male or female. Another group was asked to sort the photos only by age. The second part of the experiment tested whether the group primed to think about the photographed individuals in terms of complex identities manifested the same elderly stereotype as the group primed to think only about age. The results were striking. "When mindfulness is experimentally induced," the study's authors concluded, "it can prevent automatic stereotype-activated behavior." Mindfulness, they wrote, provides "a natural interruption in the cycle of stereotyped behavior."[14]

Medical educators whose goal is to reduce disparities have been drawing lessons from these and similar studies in cognitive psychology. Doctors' training, as one influential paper put it, should "promote the cognitive strategy of *individuation,* in which the provider focuses on the individual attributes of a particular patient, as opposed to *categorization,* in which the provider sees the patient through the filter of his or her group membership" (for example, race or age).[15] At the same time, Dr. Diana Burgess and the paper's other authors acknowledge that biases themselves are extraordinarily difficult to change. In this, they are in accord with most cognitive scientists, who argue that stereotypes are automatic and deeply ingrained, but also that they are amenable to control. Effective individuation, they say, does not eliminate a stereotype, but it does make the stereotype lose its dominant significance.[16]

We all know this ourselves. Each of us—those who are egalitarian as well as those who are overtly prejudiced—is aware of the stereotypes prevalent in our culture. There is little or perhaps nothing we can do to keep them out of our mental landscape. I am African American, and, like all African Americans, I know what the stereotypes are. But though I know what they are, they do not affect my judgment of African American individuals. Why is that? It's partly because I was taught from childhood to reject them as insulting falsifications. But it is also because I know many black people and I know that as individuals they vary in more ways than I could ever describe or enumerate. And that persuades me that the stereotypes are distortions of reality. Because I am persuaded of that, I regard the African Americans I meet as individuals rather than types. In Dr. Burgess's terms, I individuate them. And that allows me not to make the stereotypes in my head disappear but to counteract them, in a sense to neutralize them.

One effect of both cultural competence and self-awareness training is to make biases evident. Stereotypes are automatic responses. As we have seen, the biases they generate often act below the level of consciousness and influence our thinking in ways we are unaware of—in our diagnoses and treatments, if we are doctors. But once we do bring them out into the open we have the ability to deal with them. If we recognize what they are we can arm ourselves against them.

Often when I talk with doctors about health-care disparities, the immediate response is, "Not me. I treat all my patients equally. I give all of them the best care I can." "That's wonderful," I say. "I'm sure you do. But the statistics have to be coming from somewhere." If we understand our prejudices and face them honestly we can overcome them, instead of allowing them to continue overcoming us. Bringing appropriate education to bear in medical schools and ongoing professional training—that is, culturally competent care and self-awareness education—will help us to do exactly that.

Cultural competence and self-awareness training are two powerful tools we can use to break down biases, foster better doctor-patient communication, and move toward injecting equality into our unequal system of care. Another is to do everything we can to increase the number of minority physicians.

There are two reasons this is crucial. The first is that the more diversity we have among medical school classmates and faculty, the better equipped emerging doctors will be to care for minority patients. This by itself would go a long way toward reducing disparities. As I tell my students, diversity integrates the intellectual ghetto of ethnocentrism. By this I mean we all limit ourselves through our own ethnocentrism, but a diverse ecology allows for healthy, progressive penetration of our biases through integration and exposure. As Supreme Court justice Lewis Powell put it in his *Bakke* case opinion, students from diverse backgrounds "may bring to a professional school of medicine experiences, outlooks, and ideas that enrich the training of its student body and better equip its graduates to render with understanding their vital service to humanity."

A study of medical students at the University of San Francisco and Harvard made it clear that by overwhelming majorities, students themselves understand this to be true. Being members of diverse student bodies challenged them to rethink values, improved the level of classroom discussions, and more effectively prepared them, they felt, to practice medicine in a diverse society. Interestingly, those sentiments were true for students of all ethnicities, blacks, Hispanics, and Asians, as well as whites.[17]

Diversity among students and faculty naturally strengthens cultural competence. But it's not just a matter of the positive effects of interrelationships, collegiality, and exposure that are important here. Minority doctors are far more likely than mainstream doctors to work in minority neighborhoods and provide care for underserved groups. But relative to America's rapidly increasing minority population, the number of minority physicians is actually shrinking rather than growing.

Between 1980 and 2000 America's minority population grew eleven times as rapidly as the white non-Hispanic population.[18] Minorities today constitute about one-third of our population. By midcentury the Census Bureau estimates that more than half of all Americans will be from what we think of today as minority groups. At the same time, only 6 percent of the nation's physicians are African American and Hispanic, and these minorities make up only a little over 4 percent of the nation's medical school faculties.[19] The Sullivan Commission on Diversity in the Healthcare Workforce entitled its landmark 2004 report *Missing Persons: Minorities in the Health*

Professions, highlighting this massive shortage of minority medical practitioners and its impact on health care in minority communities. Sullivan and his colleagues concluded that the crisis in numbers "may be an even greater cause of disparities in health care access and outcomes than the . . . lack of health insurance for tens of millions of Americans."[20]

As chair of the Culturally Competent Care Committee, I had the visibility to push our agenda. Sitting in on many of the medical school's other committees gave me additional forums to air the views and reforms we were proposing, which I wasn't shy about doing. If I'm here, I thought, I'm here for a reason. So I spoke up.

I think that very few faculty or administrators at Harvard questioned the desirability of diversity at the medical school, and most supported at least the ideals of cultural competence and self-awareness. I knew I was in a positive environment and I was grateful for it. Dean of Faculty Joe Martin was especially supportive. He formally endorsed the need for culturally competent care and thanked me for the work we were doing. I'd hear the same kind of thing from many of my colleagues, quite a few of whom were themselves volunteering for committee work. But even with that, I was aware I was causing more than a little irritation.

I was advocating for diversity and equality, which warranted the strongest arguments I could make, and I took advantage of every opportunity. I'd hear, "Okay, culturally competent care is important. But how important? What kind of priority do you think it should have?" "Give it the physiology test," I'd answer. "How important do you feel learning physiology is to medical students? Culturally competent care has the same importance." I tried always to think of myself as a good citizen, working broadly for the medical school's betterment. But I was sure that at least some people considered me a kind of overly aggressive one-trick pony.

To a certain extent, of course, it was true. Even though I was diligently addressing a host of issues along with my committee colleagues, as often as not I would find myself prefacing my remarks at meetings with, "At the risk of being poor Johnny one-note . . . ," then I'd go on to argue my point. And all the while I was keeping my antennae out for when and to what degree I might have been creating ill will and pushback. To what extent was I overstating or being too combative?

My being African American made the dynamics more complicated than they might have been otherwise. I was antagonizing at least some of the establishment; I could just feel that. But when I talked to people, and when they talked to me, they seemed to feel obliged not to express that. To the contrary, they felt they needed to say positive things—because that was the politically correct thing to do. I had the sense that people were hypersensitive to saying something to a black professor that might be deemed overly critical, at least about diversity and disparity issues. I knew that many of my colleagues were truly with me, but others probably just appeared to be. And I couldn't always know exactly who was who.

I remembered that in New Haven, at one point there had been a black activist who somehow had gotten himself invited to participate in various deans' meetings called to talk about Yale's relations with the community. This activist was used to fighting it out in much rougher settings than these deans' affairs, and he used the vernacular fluently. At one point he was trying hard to explain, yet again, what steps the medical school ought to take to improve its standing with the African American community. He was impassioned and angry. He was telling them for the umpteenth time, You have to do this, that, and the other, but—he broke down in frustration—"but you motherfuckers aren't going to do a single one of them, are you?" I wasn't there, and nobody recorded the deans' reaction to this flagrant violation of Ivy League decorum. Personally, I tried never to be anything but dignified and respectful, no matter how hard I was arguing. But for some people, at some level, consciously or subconsciously, I was that brother and that was what they were hearing.

I knew I was pressing hard. But I also knew I was engaged in an uphill battle, that the vast weight of institutional inertia militated against the kind of approach I was advocating. Typically, a committee might meet on Monday and decide to take various steps related to diversity or cultural competence. Then we'd meet again the next week to move ahead on the committee's whole agenda, and when we were ready to adjourn nothing would have been said about the steps we had discussed the previous Monday. I'd say, "Wait a minute. What about our decision to do such and such?" There was nothing malicious about what was happening, it was just institutional inertia. The committee had a lot of issues to deal with, and diversity or cultural competence had a tendency to just float off the radar screen.

That happened again and again, and I would point it out. I advocated like mad to put culturally competent care and self-awareness into the curriculum. These seemed to me so fundamental and so intertwined that I allocated funds out of the Culturally Competent Care Committee to support the self-awareness course. I thought that Roxana and Dan's course should be mandatory for students and should be regarded as a uniquely beneficial enrichment/professional training course for faculty. I pushed hard for its inclusion and I joined the course's faculty myself. I thought Harvard should pioneer this approach and offer it for consideration as a model for other leading medical schools.

Culturally competent care, I believed, could most effectively be taught by embedding cultural awareness into the ongoing curriculum. Students learning to present cases, for example, should be taught to delineate cultural and social factors that bear on a patient's illness right along with the standard review of history, findings of the physical examination, and interpretation of lab results. Diseases such as diabetes, asthma, hypertension, and AIDS are often intertwined with the life circumstances of specific minority communities. Teaching these diseases, we believed, should extend to the racial, cultural, ethnic, and economic factors that play significant roles in the pathophysiology of the illness. Cross-cultural communication is another skill that can be taught. Students should be introduced to the problems of achieving effective rapport with patients of nonmainstream backgrounds and different linguistic capacities.

Each one of our proposals was a fight. As I write this, some have become part of Harvard's medical education and some have not. Roxana and Dan's self-awareness course no longer exists. Nevertheless, the idea of culturally competent care has made certain inroads. There are workshops, programs to prepare faculty to teach culturally competent care and others to demonstrate how to incorporate culturally competent care into standard courses—essential because we are asking faculty to teach subjects they themselves were never taught. Elements of cultural competence training have become part of some student clerkships and exam requirements.

All of these are antibias measures. They emphasize an approach that is humanistic and patient centered. They focus a doctor's attention on the patient who has a disease, as well as on the disease the patient has (to paraphrase Osler). Although patient-centered medical education and patient-centered practice have gained traction over the last number of years, it has not been a smooth path. A patient-centered orientation constitutes a significant departure from the biomedical mind-set that dominates medical education and clinical practice and that provides the main rationale for resistance to the arguments for expanding culturally competent care.

The biomedical culture, of course, stems from the prodigious and continuing advances medical science has made in understanding the causes of disease at the cellular, molecular, and genetic levels. These advances and the therapies they generate demand tremendous attention from students and clinicians, and the culture of learning and teaching that has developed around biomedicine exerts a heavy weight of inertia that naturally resists change. As Newton's first law posits, objects at rest want to stay at rest. This cultural inertia is magnified by a good measure of guilt and denial when it comes to equality issues. All together they constitute a powerful barrier to the kinds of change we were trying to bring about.

From a strictly biomedical perspective, programs such as cultural competence and self-awareness have an aura of touchy-feely fuzziness about them. To many, they seem less worthwhile than "real" medicine and have no business impinging on limited instructional time and resources. But at the same time, the arguments for expanding the teaching and practice framework to incorporate culturally competent care are hard to deny. Unequal care takes an enormous toll on the nation's health in terms of unnecessary suffering and lives lost. Several studies indicate just how enormous that toll is.

What if we were equal? That is the question several health researchers, including former surgeon general David Satcher, asked in studies that compared the number of lives saved by medical advances and the number of deaths that would have been averted if racial disparities in health care could have been resolved. Studying mortality data, researchers concluded that in the years 1991 through 2000, more than 176,000 deaths were averted through medical advances, but that correcting disparities in health care would have saved 886,000 African American lives.[21] Many of those excess African American deaths were due to disparities in access to health care and other socioeconomic factors, but prejudice in treatment, implicit and explicit, contributed its share. Inequalities in cardiac treatment, in kidney transplants, in diabetic care, and in other areas are not simply numbers and percentages on research charts. Their meaning is in lives lost and human suffering that did not have to happen.

Racial inequality has been the bane of American life in health care as elsewhere. But the same mechanisms that are behind medicine's bias regarding African Americans are at work in disparate care for other minority or "different" groups. Racism is only one of the isms we suffer from. The research literature has identified twelve groups that experience disparate care.[22] Stereotyping, poor communication, the inability or unwillingness to think beyond the purely biomedical context, the distance between doctor and patient—all these go into disparate care for women, Latinos, gays, and others. The rearrangement of the curriculum we have been working toward at Harvard, and that has become an element in other medical schools' thinking as well, seeks to enlarge the physician's scope. Cultural competence, self-awareness, communication skills, and patient-centered medicine all have one goal—humanizing the patient.

We know that well-designed training methods and pedagogies can help emerging doctors achieve a humanistic perspective on health care. But what does this mean for the day-to-day practice of medicine in emergency rooms and clinics and doctors' offices where physicians encounter patients from backgrounds as diverse as our pluralistic society has to offer?

What it means is nothing less than a reorientation in the physician's perspective on what he is supposed to be doing. It means an expansion in physicians' understanding of what standard care ought to be. "Humanizing the patient" sounds like a positive, liberal concept, easy to embrace. But practicing humanistic medicine requires real, often time-consuming investments. It asks doctors to make what they might initially think of as extra effort, but which should actually be considered part and parcel of normal practice.

Humanistic medical practice breaks into two parts. One might be called the *organization* of care. This encompasses practices that contribute to building trust—which initiates the pathway of effective communication, patient satisfaction, adherence to therapeutic regimens, and better outcomes. It also includes awareness of the patient's circumstances—his or her ability to fulfill the requirements of treatment. The second might be called the *spirit* of care. This applies to the mind-set of physicians as they interact with patients.

The Organization of Humanistic Care

A patient's visit begins when she enters the doctor's office or clinic. What is there in the office that indicates the doctor's affiliation with this patient? If the practice serves African Americans or Latinos, are there photographs or pictures that suggest the doctor's interest and concern? Are there appropriate magazines and other reading material? Is there a person of color or common ethnic affiliation to greet the patient? Are the reception personnel trained to anticipate and help with problems regarding insurance and other paperwork? Is there help for patients with poor health literacy or low English-language proficiency?

In the examination room, has the physician taken steps to examine patients from cultures that may have strict modesty customs with appropriate respect and sensitivity? Is a translator available if necessary? Has the physician developed techniques for making certain that patients understand prescriptions or other treatment regimens?

Is the physician sufficiently familiar with the patient's life circumstances to know if he will be able to get prescriptions filled? Many pharmacies in African American neighborhoods, for example, do not stock certain analgesics. If a follow-up visit is important, does the physician know how difficult it might be for the patient to take time off from work? Has the physician taken steps to accommodate patients who might need to make a follow-up telephone call but cannot communicate well in English? Patients' limitations in areas such as these will affect their ability to adhere to therapies. For minorities and patients from lower socioeconomic groups, physicians should be able to anticipate potential difficulties and provide guidance and, when necessary, advocacy.

The Spirit of Humanistic Care

In the previous chapter I mentioned Dr. Joseph Betancourt, the professor of health policy at Massachusetts General Hospital. Though I quoted him earlier, I think it's worthwhile reiterating here his comment that, deeply ingrained in our medical culture, "there is almost a built-in good patient/bad patient [distinction]. The bad patient being the one where you have to take extra steps to sort things out."

That bad patient is almost always the elderly patient, the black or Hispanic or gay or obese or disabled patient, the clinic patient as opposed to the private patient. (As one of my colleagues puts it, "As soon as you say 'private patient'/'clinic patient' you are dealing in disparity. Just say 'patient.'")[23] That bad patient is exactly the patient who is on the receiving end of disparate care.

Humanistic medicine asks the physician to organize her practice around an awareness of that patient's needs. But it also challenges the physician to undertake a further and more difficult effort— this one directed inward.

The fundamental requirement of humanistic medicine is openness to recognizing our own biases and the desire to counteract them. Humanistic, or egalitarian, medicine asks us to candidly assess some of our most private and least acknowledged attitudes. Do we at some deep level, aside from what may be our liberal professions, think of African Americans as intellectually or morally inferior? Do we regard women as fragile physically and more vulnerable emotionally? Do we believe that the lives of the elderly are worth less than the lives of younger people? Do we think of Latino and other immigrants as difficult strangers with alien values? Do we regard the obese with distaste and aversion? Whether or not we have gay friends, do we at heart view homosexuality as troubling and abnormal?

If we are honest, many of us might own up to at least some feelings of this sort. Lay people with a regard for equality might simply ignore or suppress such biases, never having to actively deal with them. Physicians, though, bear a special humanistic and egalitarian obligation. We have undertaken to heal our fellow human beings. And because we now are fully aware of the impact bias and prejudice have on the delivery of health care, and because we have come to understand the immense cost of unequal treatment, we, unlike lay people, are under a powerful moral imperative to actively confront our biases in order to ensure that they do not continue to affect the work we have set for ourselves.

That is a hard psychological challenge, particularly because our training in most cases is focused elsewhere. But we should know that the process carries with it immense personal as well as professional rewards. In practicing humanistic medicine, we fulfill ourselves as physicians as we would not otherwise. To the extent that we recognize the worth and validity of our patients, they offer us in exchange the gift of recognizing our own humanity, expressed in trust, in confidence, and in satisfaction with us as healers. It is a kind of reciprocal blessing.

A variety of contemporary stressors make doctors' lives difficult—the pressures to see and take care of more patients faster, the mounting financial and time-consuming burdens of paperwork, the fear of legal suits and growing insurance costs, the ever-quickening pace of medical discoveries that we must try to keep up with. The bottom line is that many doctors see the practice of medicine as a less and less satisfying pursuit, more like a business and increasingly impersonal. A growing body of literature describes this disturbing increase in physician distress and burnout.[24] But the heart of medical practice is still that intimate encounter between the physician and the patient. To make that encounter successful, physicians need to close the distance that always exists between individuals and that widens with differences in race, in gender, in ethnicity, in language. Success in that endeavor adds greatly to the doctor's satisfaction with what he does. In the face of all the stressors, it goes a long way toward making the work worthwhile.

It was Montague Cobb, the great African American anatomist, medical anthropologist, and civil rights leader, who used the expression "My fellow humans" to begin his speeches. I took it from him after hearing him lecture at Yale, where I had invited him to speak. I was drawn to the phrase then as a striking way of expressing fellowship with an audience. But as the years have passed, I have come to understand it more fully. I think now that Cobb was not just greeting an audience, I think he was extending an invitation to them. In calling them his fellow humans, he expected that they would return the favor. That was something, in those days, for a black American to say to a white audience. Times have changed considerably since then. But the essential message of the phrase hasn't. To the extent we recognize the humanity of those different from us, to that extent will they recognize us as their own fellow humans, as part of their own large family. And in taking this step, I think Cobb would say, we enlarge not only them but ourselves as well.

EPILOGUE

We understand that medicine is a science. We are less aware that it is also an art. And art, we know, depends upon the humanity of the artist.

—Memphis Slim

IN FEBRUARY 2009 the *New York Post* published a cartoon. Two policemen, one with a smoking gun in his hand, are standing in front of the bullet-riddled body of a dead chimpanzee. One policeman says to the other, "They'll have to find someone else to write the next stimulus bill." After a few months, not many recalled the dreadful story of a pet chimpanzee that had run amok in Stamford, Connecticut, badly injured a woman, and was shot by police—the news item alluded to by the cartoon. But the depiction of President Obama as a chimpanzee stayed in people's minds.

The reason it did was that the historical association of blacks with apes is so deeply ingrained in the national consciousness.[1] In Europe it's common for soccer fans to make monkey noises at black players and throw bananas. While that kind of public display wouldn't be tolerated in America, during the 2008 presidential campaign, Internet portrayals of then candidate Obama as a monkey proliferated.

Linking blacks with apes has always been an insidious dehumanizing mechanism, nurturing a mind-set that African Americans are an inferior species, not meriting the same rights, opportunities, and consideration as real (that is, white) human beings. And yet Barack Obama was elected president because a large percentage of white Americans as well as African Americans considered him the better man to lead the nation in a time of crisis. Clearly, in some ways we as a society have evolved past our racist heritage. But at the same time, deep-set conceptions of racial superiority and inferiority persist. As a people, we carry our commitment to equality right alongside a collection of what I have called in this book *isms*—racism, sexism, ageism, and other isms—prejudices that have real-life consequences, most particularly in medicine.

These isms are crystallized in stereotypes we cannot help but harbor—whether we accept them or not—because they reflect ingrained cultural attitudes. Attitudes of this sort build themselves into the culture over long expanses of time. By the same token, they lose their grasp only gradually in the face of changing perceptions, and they can put up a fierce rear-guard defense of their hold on people's minds. In a way, that is how I've seen the context of efforts, mine and others', to change the conception of how medicine should be taught and how patients should be treated. Culturally competent care and cultural self-awareness are part of a struggle against entrenched prejudices and stereotypes that hold on tenaciously, their grip measured in the grim statistics of unequal treatment.

But medicine has never been an isolated endeavor. The circumstances of the larger society's life are also medicine's circumstances. The perceptions that govern doctor-patient relationships are not different from those that mediate relationships more generally. Equal treatment in medicine makes progress only as physicians shed their biases; the same holds true for the larger world of which medicine is a part.

At a meeting for fellows in a Harvard administrative program a number of years ago, I found myself sitting at a table alongside then president Larry Summers. During our conversation together we talked for a while about medicine, and I was struck by his indepth knowledge of science. Scientific literacy was, he said, essential to living life intelligently. That's right, I thought. Scientific literacy—and also cultural literacy.

Of course, I was engaged full time with issues of cultural competence in medicine, so the idea that cultural literacy might be an essential element of education generally wasn't that much of a stretch. But a recent news item that bore on this subject had caught my attention, and I had also just seen a movie that I thought spoke powerfully about the perils inherent in cultural *il*literacy.

The news item came from Argentina. A Brazilian handyman there had confessed to the brutal bludgeoning murder of an American oil executive and his wife. The murder, and now the confession, had drawn international attention, not just because the murdered man had been an important industrial figure, but because he and his wife were white while the Brazilian handyman was black. In his confession, the handyman said that the executive had called him "the worst racial slur, in fluent Portuguese."

The movie was *Crash,* which won the best-picture Oscar in 2005. *Crash* was about the destructive stereotypes we carry with us. It depicts how these can create havoc and violence in a heartbeat. It is also full of constant surprises that turn these stereotypes on their heads and reveal, as often as not, the underlying humanity of the film's characters.

There's nothing new about race-motivated violence, but the Argentine murder was a stark example of both the ignorance and the depth of feeling that go into it. I had been through Roxana and Dan's cultural awareness course several years earlier and was now helping to teach it. If any of those three people, I thought, had taken the course, or anything like it, the incident never would have happened. Likewise, the movie portrayed how we, in our different groups, misconstrue one another without seeing the essential things that bind us together. What a dramatic presentation of exactly the themes Dan, Roxana, I, and our other faculty members were focusing on.

Cultural literacy, I began to think, isn't needed only in the doctor-patient relationship. Cross-cultural ignorance and misunderstanding in any setting can be rough, embarrassing, even fatal. Cross-cultural skills are a day-to-day requirement for most of us, for how we function in the normal course of our lives. Some people are intuitively good at this—our pediatrician friend Joe Kramer, for instance, who cared for families on New York's multiethnic Lower East

Side. Then there are the others, who need some kind of intervention to stimulate their awareness. And it became obvious to me at some point that cultural literacy should be included in our basic education. Larry Summers had said that scientific literacy was a requirement for living intelligently; how much more so, then, is an understanding of what it takes to function harmoniously with those of other cultures, with whom we mix as co-workers, clients, acquaintances, friends, patients, or just ordinary fellow citizens. And what better way to do it than in Roxana and Dan's course, or some iteration of that?

Cultural literacy, from that point of view, is complementary to the cultural literacy that scholars in the humanities talk about, which constitutes much of the core curriculum at many American colleges and universities.[2] Almost everyone with a college education has been exposed to at least some of the fundamental elements of Western culture, to the religious and intellectual developments, to the history, the politics, the philosophy, the literature and arts that have gone into forming something that might be called the common cultural identity of those of us, at least, who make our lives here.

Unfortunately, the dominant culture has historically brought with it a disregard and derogation of groups that are outside the mainstream. But there's no logical reason a grounding in the general culture should necessitate a lack of respect for or devaluing of the various distinct cultures that are the heritage of our varied population. Nor does embracing our various distinct ethnic cultures necessarily imply any rejection of the common culture we do share. Our individual cultures must be valued and affirmed. That is the pluralist ideal. But we can enjoy and celebrate our distinct cultural identities without sacrificing our common bonds, just as we can celebrate the elements of our common identity without giving up our distinctiveness. Pluralism should lead to community. Community should embrace pluralism. That is the ultimate goal of a diverse society like ours.

The traditional, humanistic kind of cultural literacy is learning driven. Its purpose is to deepen our understanding of the historical forces that have contributed to making us who we are intellectually, morally, and spiritually. The cross-cultural literacy that our self-awareness faculty was teaching is pragmatic. Its aim is to better understand ourselves so that we can better understand and empathize with others.

The doctor-patient interaction is perhaps the paradigm of pragmatic relationships. It has a specific purpose and a desired outcome. In medicine, cross-cultural literacy improves health outcomes. But self-awareness and cross-cultural literacy for nondoctors is pragmatic as well. Its purpose is more diffuse but equally goal oriented. It is to bind us together as a community. It is to teach us how to better succeed in a nation—and a world—replete with varieties of peoples and cultures. We are part, after all, of a global community that needs cross-cultural literacy at least as desperately as we need it here at home. The progression I had envisioned all the way back when our visiting committee was reporting on diversity at Brown University was "diversity to pluralism to community"; *Diversity, Pluralism and Community* was, in fact, the title of our second report. Back then our fundamental question was: How can we best validate and dignify our diverse cultures, and nurture their interaction so that our overall community is enriched and strengthened? Now I thought I was seeing more clearly how those particular dots connected.

With that I began to push forward with the idea that cross-cultural literacy and cultural awareness should be part of all students' education. I talked with colleagues whenever I had a chance and I developed a more formal presentation. I found there was already something of a movement along those lines, which confirmed my conviction that understanding ourselves in relation to others, especially "different" others, should be an essential element in everyone's education, as it should be in everyone's toolbox of survival skills.[3] I spoke with Ruth Simmons, president of Brown; Steve Hyman, Harvard's provost; Evelyn Hammonds, Harvard's dean of arts and sciences; with the advisory board of Stanford's Center for Comparative Studies in Race and Ethnicity; to colleagues at the University of Mississippi and Vanderbilt University. In various places I've pre-cipitated discussions about starting out by making cultural literacy a premed requirement, and I have proposed that to the American Association of Medical Colleges.

The right kind of education can be a powerful instrument in moving us toward equality. But there's no substitute for the effect of real-life exposure to the thoughts, perspectives, and world views of those who are not members of our own immediate group. Exposure of that sort expands our reach; it stretches our own way of perceiv-ing and thinking. It magnifies our intellectual and moral firepower.

But in order for our institutions to reach a meaningful level of diversity, minorities first have to get a seat at the table. Through most of my own life and career, African Americans had no seat at the table, which I felt keenly. But then, neither did Latinos or women, let alone other disadvantaged minorities. Louis Sullivan and Alvin Poussaint are the same age, which is more or less my age too. They were both residents at Cornell Medical Center in New York, though they had never met before. One day on the ward, Poussaint spotted Sullivan and went over to introduce himself. Sullivan looked up in surprise and said, "What in the world are you doing here?" I don't know what I would have said had I suddenly come across another African American intern or resident. Probably the same thing.

There was a saying in the South when I was growing up, some-thing parents and teachers used to tell children: "You can't just be as good as whites, you have to be twice as good." That was a spur to work harder, because if you were only "as good," you'd never have a chance against white kids. There are, of course, some blacks who are "twice as good," not just at the very top vis-à-vis whites, but at the top vis-à-vis anyone. I'm thinking, for example, of Martin Luther King or Barack Obama or Muhammad Ali. But if we are going to achieve any meaningful diversity we can't wait for the the Martins, Baracks, and Muhammads. We have to bring along minorities who are merely "as good" as the competition.

The challenge is doing that in the face of the racism that characterized and still does characterize our economy, our educational system, and our institutions. Institutionalized racism and other "isms" keep doors closed to minorities through custom and practice.[4] Sandra Day O'Connor, for example, graduated number three in her Stanford Law School class—in two years rather than the customary three—yet the only job she was offered in California was as a legal secretary. Ruth Bader Ginsburg graduated number one from Columbia Law School, but had an equivalent experience in New York. Custom in those years kept the doors firmly shut against women lawyers.

Here's how institutionalized racism worked at Harvard Medical School. In 1968 African American enrollment at all American medical schools other than Howard and Meharry totaled 133. That's 133 in the entire country. In other words, the doors were shut—other than for a tiny handful of us who somehow managed to squeeze our way in. But on April 4 of that year, Martin Luther King was assassinated, which led to a countrywide crisis, including some substantial soul searching on the part of whites. Three days after the assassination an ad hoc group of nine Harvard medical school faculty members started work on a resolution that called for affirmative action. They proposed that fifteen "Negroes" should be admitted each year rather than the three or fewer that was customary.

Given the trauma of the King assassination, there was no outright opposition. But some were skeptical that Harvard could find fifteen qualified African Americans. Let's be clear on what that meant. It meant that in 1968 some Harvard Medical School faculty did not believe that in the entire United States there were fifteen African Americans intelligent and hard working enough to be successful HMS students. Other faculty resisted the proposal because they thought "quotas" were wrong. This in spite of the fact that African Americans had historically been subject to the very harshest of educational institution admissions quotas, allowing only small numbers (in my day Brown generally took five per class) or, most frequently, no numbers at all.

The ad hoc group's resolution passed, but only after a compromise was reached that the school would increase the size of its entering class from 125 to 140. In other words, it took something as cataclysmic as Dr. King's death to spring open Harvard Medical School's admissions, and even then it was a fight.[5]

At Harvard it was affirmative action that wedged those doors open. Affirmative action has done that; it has pried doors open around the country, and kept them open. Justice Powell in his *Bakke* decision declared that diversity enriches a student body. Sandra Day O'Connor echoed Powell's opinion in the University of Michigan Law School case *(Grutter v. Bollinger)* that challenged affirmative action in the Supreme Court and lost. She wrote of the "compelling interest" of the law school in achieving a diverse student body, that "diversity promotes learning outcomes and better prepares students for an increasingly diverse workforce and society." She quoted the United States government *amicus curiae* brief and concluded that "effective participation by members of all racial and ethnic groups in the civic life of our Nation is essential if the dream of one Nation, indivisible, is to be realized."

The American Academy of Orthopedic Surgeons was one of many *amici* supporting affirmative action in the Michigan case. I had had the opportunity to weigh in on the orthopedic surgeons' decision to do that. In my presentation in front of the board of directors, I addressed the often-heard criticism that affirmative action elevates the unqualified at the expense of the qualified. Major studies have given the lie to that canard. The largest, by Derek Bok (Harvard's long-term president) and William Bowen (past president of Princeton), studied 45,000 students who had been admitted to elite American colleges over a twenty-year period. Comparing those admitted via affirmative action to those admitted under normal procedures, they found that regularly admitted students got better grades and graduated at a higher rate, but that affirmative action students entered medical, law, business, and other graduate schools at a higher rate and were more active in civic affairs.[6] A similar long-term study of medical students at the University of California–Davis showed that while regularly admitted students had a slightly higher graduation rate (97 percent as opposed to 94 percent), there was no difference between the groups regarding specialization rates, performance as residents, or honors received. There was "no evidence," the authors concluded, "of diluting the quality of the graduates."[7]

Far from being some kind of vehicle for incorporating inferiority into our institutions, affirmative action is a mechanism for making the invisible visible, for bringing attention to talented minority students who would otherwise remain unnoticed. That was certainly my experience on Yale Medical School's admissions committee and on the Harvard Combined Orthopedic Program executive committee. Some, at least, of those minority students and trainees who were admitted during my tenure would not have been noticed had I or someone like me not been there to push for them. That was affirmative action in a small sphere. I was fortunate to be at the table in those places (together with Jim Comer at Yale). If some minority member had not been, the dead hand of institutional inertia and customary racial discrimination would have kept its iron grip on those procedures.

There's a story about Colin Powell that's relevant here. During the Jimmy Carter administration an African American, Clifford Alexander, was secretary of the army. One of the secretary's duties is to select officers for promotion to the rank of general from a list provided through the service's normal promotion channels. When that list was brought to Alexander, he asked the colonel who presented it how many minority candidates it included. Taken aback, the colonel told Alexander he wasn't sure, he'd have to check. When he did, it turned out that there weren't any. "Do you mean to tell me," Alexander said, "that in the whole United States Army there are no minority officers eligible for promotion to general officer?" The colonel left, shamefaced, and returned with an augmented list that included Colin Powell's name, which Alexander duly selected. Of course, Powell rose from there to become chairman of the Joint Chiefs of Staff, national security advisor, and secretary of state. That was affirmative action at work as well—making the invisible Colonel Powell into the visible General Powell.

Writing about President Obama's nomination of Sonia Sotomayor to the Supreme Court, *New York Times* legal columnist Adam

Liptak described how the mere presence of a minority member alters the dynamic of a court. Even conservative justices acknowledge that Thurgood Marshall, for example, "exerted a gravitational pull" that went far beyond the power of his one vote. "Marshall could be a persuasive presence just by sitting there," said Justice Scalia. "He wouldn't have to open his mouth to affect the nature of the conference and how seriously the conference would take matters of race."[8] Sotomayor's impact on the Supreme Court will no doubt turn out to be similar—she brings a perspective informed by a Hispanic woman's life experiences. Her very presence creates an effect.

We are still reaching in so many of our institutions for that equalizing presence. That's not to say, of course, that we haven't made progress. In the medical world, even though the number of blacks in influential roles is limited, it is, at least, no longer nonexistent. Don Wilson was long-term dean at the University of Maryland Medical School. Roy Wilson is chancellor of the University of Colorado, including its medical school. Cato Laurencin is vice president for health affairs at the University of Connecticut and dean of the university's medical school. Tony Rankin is a recent president of the American Academy of Orthopedic Surgeons. John Ruffin is director of the NIH's Institute of Minority Health and Health Disparities. JudyAnn Bigby is the Massachusetts secretary for health and human services. At my own institution, Nancy Oriol is dean of students, Joan Reede is dean for diversity, and Alvin Poussaint is associate dean for student affairs. There are others of us playing leading roles in the American health establishment as well. With all that, though, we, like other minorities, are still painfully underrepresented.

At one point in my career I was tapped for a senior position as well. It was a brief but instructive experience. In 1989, while I was chief of orthopedics at Beth Israel, the University of Maryland at Baltimore was searching for a new president. The university consisted of seven graduate schools—medicine, law, social work, dentistry, nursing, pharmacy, and arts and sciences—all located centrally in Baltimore's inner city, with its large African American population. One of the search committee's criteria was apparently to find someone who could promote closer ties between the university and its surrounding community, and my name had been submitted by then Secretary of Health and Human Services Lou Sullivan.

In the course of various interviews it became clear that the search committee was seriously interested in nominating me. After a lot of thought, I had concluded that if they did want me, I would do it. This was an opportunity to assume a major leadership role of an unusual institution with great interdisciplinary potential. It would mean giving up my surgical career, which I loved, but in return I would have the opportunity to make an impact across a range of health and human service disciplines, as well as to play a significant role in the Greater Baltimore community. By the middle of June the search committee decided to appoint me, and I enthusiastically accepted.

Two months later, before I had even taken office, I handed the chancellor my resignation. It was a particularly hard decision, but unavoidable, I thought. What had happened was that a few days earlier the chairman of the Board of Regents had abruptly informed me that the law school and the school of social work would be removed administratively from the university at Baltimore and relocated outside of the city. I had been talking and negotiating about the presidency of seven schools; now the seven were suddenly reduced to five. Just as significantly, the two that were to be removed—law and social work—provided extensive services and programs for the city's minority community. It was, I thought, a truly awful decision.

Beyond that, I, as the incoming president, had been neither consulted nor even informed. That was stunning. They wanted me, yet it was clear they had little respect for either me, the office, or the institution. It was doubly clear that they had little or no regard for the community from which they were about to strip a host of essential services, not to mention jobs. I didn't know how much, if any, of this had a racial component to it, but when I reflected on it later on I thought it might well have had. I did know that this wasn't an environment I could work in.

I was sorry this had happened. I saw the university as a diamond in the rough. Moreover, I thought I had a chance here to forge an especially creative and mutually beneficial relationship between the university and the community. Of course, for me personally it wasn't a disaster; I was going back to my operating room, which in any event had been difficult to give up. But my whole career had been teaching me the lesson that in order to break the hold of racism, we needed a seat at the table, and that would have been an important seat. At the time there were only one or two black presidents of large mainstream universities, and this was a consortium of graduate schools right next to the power centers of Washington, in a city with a black mayor, Kurt Schmoke, and a vibrant black population, which I was already getting to know. So from that point of view too I was particularly saddened that it didn't work out.

It also reinforced for me the truth that the endeavor of African Americans and other minorities to make an equal place for themselves in American life is a long march if there ever was one. Even now, with Barack Obama as president, we are far from being out of the woods. In Sandra Day O'Connor's Michigan decision she noted that it might be twenty-five years before we can do without affirmative action. If only. The fact is that we had almost four hundred years of slavery, apartheid, and de jure and de facto discrimination to get racism embedded in our system. How long it might take to get it out is an open question.

To make equality real, then—not just for African Americans but also for women, Hispanics, and other minorities—institutions have to seriously commit themselves to diversity as a critical priority. They have to come to the challenge knowing that they—every major hospital, college, professional school, union, and business—were founded by white males to serve a white male-dominated culture. Changing the culture of those institutions takes determination and the willpower to stay the course, however long that course may be. "Without struggle," as Frederick Douglass said, "there is no progress."[9]

As minorities come into our institutions in leadership roles, the inbred psychology of prejudice will erode over time. To some degree it has already. It will continue to do so. Other forces also contribute to the process. In his book *Privilege, Power, and Difference*, sociologist Allan Johnson describes the effect of individuals taking small steps to bring about change in their own spheres of influence. "You don't have to do anything dramatic or earth-shaking to help change happen," he says. "As powerful as systems of privilege are, they cannot stand the strain of lots of people doing something about it."[10] In the medical world, it isn't necessary to wait for global changes in education or new health legislation in order for doctors to make changes in how they conduct their own practices. When I discuss these subjects with peers, I often say that at bottom, to significantly diminish disparities in health care all we really need to do is treat all our patients as if they were family or friends. That's something we can all accomplish within our own spheres. It may not address the complexities of unequal treatment, but it is a powerful and doable first step.

I don't believe that simple appeal—to treat patients like family and friends—is completely naïve. The reason I don't think so is that, in fact, a physician's work is humanitarian at its core. In practicing modern medicine, permeated as it is with sophisticated science, elaborate tests, and high-tech devices and procedures, it's easy to lose sight of the fact that patient care means care of the patient. But what is a doctor's function? What is it that they actually do? The answer is that doctors heal their fellow human beings. Physicians may be scientists, statisticians, device makers, high-level technicians, but in essence they are human beings who take care of other human beings. And these other human beings they care for—all are, to one degree or another, strangers. And that—caring for strangers as if they were your own—is, I think, as good a definition as one could give of what it means to be a humanitarian.

In that way doctoring is, perhaps, *the* paradigmatic humanitarian profession. Because it is, doctors should by rights see themselves—and they should be seen by others—as humanitarian role models. And that is one reason unequal health care is so corrosive to society's values. Not only is disparate care profoundly unjust, its injustice is carried out by a profession that should be a leading exemplar of the egalitarian and humanitarian spirit.

In my own life in medicine I have been a clinician, a scientist, and an educator. My homes have been the doctor's office and the university. In considering how to cut the Gordian knot of disparate care, the hopes I have center on these two settings.

First, I would like to leave a strong hope and challenge to medical schools. I believe it's incumbent on them to strategically direct energy and resources toward developing the humanitarian, patient-centered, culturally competent aspects of medicine and to institutionalize this direction as a mainstream goal, to make it more than a half-hearted acknowledgment or afterthought and pursue it as a core mission, equal in importance to other important missions of the schools. We have till now gestured toward and toyed with these concepts, but we have not forcefully resolved, with the required resources, determination, and commitment, to give humane medicine a substantial role in our leading medical schools.

Second, for the practicing physician. We all know that many, if not most, students arrive in medical school imbued with idealism and a sense of humane purpose. We most likely came in that way ourselves. But all too often that humane purpose gets diluted along the way. It gets lost among the pressures and rigors of training, among the conditioning effects of the biomedical culture. It is assaulted by the callousness of the informal curriculum we pick up in the hallways and from some of our teachers and supervisors. It recedes before the mountain of debt we incur for our education.

But practicing medicine is something that should allow us to keep in close touch with our ideals; it should appeal day in and day out to the satisfaction and pleasure that we expected to get out of being a doctor. I don't know how many doctors experience this or don't experience it. But I can tell you that I don't think it's part of the culture. I think the culture tends to downplay the joy of fixing something that's wrong, of helping the patient. I know that when I've emphasized this in professional meetings I've felt like I was pointing up something that's not quite within the approved guidelines. But it should be. Give yourself a chance to be fulfilled by what you are doing. Seize on that. It's okay. Seize on it and appreciate it.

That's really what humanitarian medicine—egalitarian medicine—is about. Its key words are empathy, cooperation, and communication. Humanitarian medicine is what I like to call win, win, win. The patient wins. The doctor wins. The society wins in improving the health of the whole population, minority as well as mainstream. It wins for us all in a larger sense too, in providing a model for the spirit of community and mutual care that we so urgently need, and so lack, in our increasingly splintered and sectarian world.

SOME PRACTICAL SUGGESTIONS FOR PATIENTS AND PHYSICIANS

Following are some practical suggestions for patients and physicians meant to heighten awareness of cultural issues and enhance the delivery of quality, nondiscriminatory medical treatment.

FOR PATIENTS

The bottom line for patients is to understand that health care is most effective when there is good communication between you and your doctor. Keep in mind that your doctor is a medical expert with many years of training, but he or she is also a human being who, like you, responds to friendliness and openness. So:

Humanize Your Doctor

Try to strike up a level of rapport. Don't be afraid to engage in small talk, about your family, the weather, whatever works to start things off on a friendly basis. People generally, minority people especially, may feel intimidated by a doctor, or uncomfortable, or even suspicious. Feelings like these may be stronger if the doctor's race, ethnicity, gender, or sexual orientation is different from yours. But half the responsibility of getting over cultural or other differences belongs to you. So build bridges any way you can, and meet your doctor halfway across them.

You may want to do a little cross-cultural homework as part of your doctor selection. What is the doctor's gender, race, ethnicity, age, and so forth—whatever might be of concern to you. Do you have friends or acquaintances who have gone to this particular doctor? What was their experience?

Whether or not you have done any homework of this kind, you may find yourself feeling uncomfortable with the doctor. Perhaps he or she seems disinterested or distant or discourteous. In that case you might try something like this:

"I came here because I know you are a good doctor. I don't want to be disrespectful, but I'd like to know if you've taken care of many Asian patients (substitute, for example, African American, Latino, Native American, Islamic). The reason I ask this is because I don't feel as though we're communicating as well as we might."

The doctor's response may be sincere and concerned or possibly even surprised. Those are good signs. They suggest he or she will make an effort to communicate better.

The doctor may try to quickly move past your concerns without engaging them. If that's the case, you have to rely on your gut feeling about what to do. Maybe this is a person you just will not be able to get along with. Or maybe you'll feel that even though this individual may lack warmth, he or she is nevertheless an excellent physician who wants to help and whom you will want to stay with.

It's also possible the doctor will react with annoyance or denial or even an element of hostility. In that case, you should find a new doctor.

Read about Your Symptoms or Disease, if You Know It

There are many reference books and an increasing number of helpful Web sites that you can go to for information. MayoClinic.com and WebMD are two popular and reliable Internet sites.

Generally, the more you know about your disease, the more you will be able to help your doctor to help you. Keep in mind that you and the doctor want to be the strongest partnership you can be against the disease—the two of you as a team. The more you know, the better questions you can ask and the more understanding you will have about your doctor's diagnosis and recommended course of treatment.

Do a "Teach Back" with Your Doctor

Even when doctors do their best to explain clearly what medication or medications you should take and when and how often you should take them, you may not understand clearly. This is especially so when there is more than one medication involved or if you are not completely fluent in English. This is why we recommend for both patients and doctors that the patient should do a "Teach Back." A Teach Back is when, after the doctor tells you what medications you should take or what other instructions you should follow, you teach them back to him. Your Teach Back might start like this: "Doctor, please let me try and tell you what I understand to see if I am completely clear about what you have told me." After you have explained to him, he will either confirm that you understand or he will go over things again. This is extremely important because following the doctor's instructions carefully is the key element to treating your disease or problem successfully.

Take a Friend or Relative into the Doctor's Office with You if You Feel You Need To

This is a good habit if you have a relative or close friend you don't mind knowing about your medical problem. Having someone with you provides additional ears, additional understanding, and additional judgment. If you have someone with you, you might feel more comfortable and have less anxiety when talking to the doctor.

FOR DOCTORS AND DOCTORS-IN-TRAINING

Have a Basic Understanding of the Cultures Your Patients Come From

Sensitivity to some basic attitudinal and behavior patterns of your patients' cultures may well assist in your effort to achieve a helpful level of rapport and communication. In some cultures, for example, patients have an exceptionally high degree of respect for doctors. Lack of openness or communication may be due to deference or feelings of intimidation or powerlessness that are stronger than what you might expect from mainstream patients. In such cases you will want to take extra care to elicit questions and identify potential misunderstanding or confusion on the patient's part. If you do make a mistake, and we all do, step back, apologize sincerely, and move on.

Cultural sensitivity can also save you from unintentional faux pas and needless misunderstandings that can start your relationship off on the wrong foot. You may, for example, be in the habit of calling your patients by their first names—or your staff might be. This may or may not be a good idea generally. It is most definitely not a good idea with African American patients, who may be especially sensitive to indications of disrespect. Another example: Recognize that certain Middle Eastern cultures have taboos about cross-gender touching or observing. Take that into account before launching into your standard examination routine.

Don't Stereotype Your Patients, Individuate Them

While a basic sensitivity toward cultural patterns can help you avoid errors, don't assume that patients conform to stereotypes. Just because a patient is a member of a particular group does not mean he or she will embody elements of any generalized stereotype. Keep in mind that stereotypes may be cultural, having to do with emotionality, intelligence, lifestyles, and so forth of different racial or ethnic groups—or they may be more strictly medical, having to do with the prevalence of certain physiological problems or syndromes among specific groups. These generalized understandings can easily lead to attributional errors. They can lead you to a particular diagnosis because the symptoms seem to fit the stereotype, when what you really need to do is keep an open mind and think outside the box. To do that we have to make the strongest effort to see each patient as an individual rather than a type.

Understand and Respect the Tremendous Power of Unconscious Bias

Keep in mind that (1) biases are often unconscious, (2) in one way or another we all have them, and (3) they can strongly influence and interfere with our communication with patients and with our diagnoses and treatments. Do everything you can to become aware of and honestly face the biases that you personally might have, both those you know you have and those that take some digging to recognize.

There are some mechanisms available to help with self-awareness, such as the Banaji Implicit Association Test, which you can take online in total privacy. But the most effective measure is our willingness to confront our deepest feelings about those who are different from us. If we do that, we can then take steps to mitigate the effects those feelings and biases have. We can plant a warning flag in our emotions that will keep us vigilant in our attempt to provide the best and most treatment to all of our patients equally. Use what I like to call the F and F approach, Friends and Family. Consciously treating all of our patients, most especially those who differ from us, as if they were friends and family will go far toward eliminating disparate treatment.

Recognize Situations That Magnify Stereotyping and Bias

Doctors frequently work under a variety of powerful stressors. There are time pressures as we are pushed to see more and more patients. In some specialties and especially as interns and residents we are often sleep deprived. Coming out of training, most young doctors are in serious debt. At the same time, it has become increasingly difficult to collect reimbursements for our services. At this writing, it costs approximately $85,000 a year for nonclinical staff in order to collect payments. Simply keeping up on significant research and advances in our own fields is a daunting challenge. One respected source figured that to do just this one thing well, internists, for example, would need to read nineteen articles a day every day of the year.

I am not mentioning these facts to bewail the physician's lot. The healer's art carries with it immense personal rewards and the irreplaceable pleasure of working at something that is not just a job but a vocation. But—stress has consequences. One of those consequences is that the more stress we are under the more we rely on shortcuts, and stereotyping is perhaps the major mental shortcut. It is precisely when we are rushed and anxious that we most need to rededicate ourselves to providing equal care.

Know the CLAS Standards

The National Standards on Culturally and Linguistically Appropriate Services (CLAS) are primarily directed at health-care organizations, but individual physicians should be familiar with them and should strive to see that they are reflected in an appropriate way in their own practices. They provide guidelines and in some cases mandates for how to make your setting comfortable and culturally competent as you serve minority patients. For your convenience we have listed these standards following this section.

Do a "Teach Back"

Patients should be educated about the importance of doing a Teach Back to make sure they understand your instructions. But many if not most will not know the technique. Be sure you do a Teach Back with them if there is any question at all that they do not completely understand the medications or other therapies you are prescribing. Be most diligent about this if your patient has limited English or comes from a culture where medical and health practices differ from ours. Don't be satisfied until you are sure the patient truly gets what you are telling him or her.

Assiduously Practice Evidence-Based Medicine

Following such protocols with all patients will greatly protect equal treatment. EBM recognizes that good medical care depends partly on individual and social factors that are not strictly subject to scientific methods. But in stressing the examination of evidence on the basis of clinical research and systematic reasoning, EBM provides a paradigm not just for excellence in treatment, but for equal treatment.

NATIONAL STANDARDS ON CULTURALLY AND LINGUISTICALLY APPROPRIATE SERVICES

The following is a list of National Standards on Culturally and Linguistically Appropriate Services (CLAS), as issued by the U.S. Department of Health and Human Services Office of Minority Health, March 2001, available at http://www.omhrc.gov/assets/pdf/checked/finalreport.pdf.

STANDARD 1

Health care organizations should ensure that patients/consumers receive from all staff members effective, understandable, and respectful care that is provided in a manner compatible with their cultural health beliefs and practices and preferred language.

STANDARD 2

Health care organizations should implement strategies to recruit, retain, and promote at all levels of the organization a diverse staff and leadership that are representative of the demographic characteristics of the service area.

STANDARD 3

Health care organizations should ensure that staff at all levels and across all disciplines receive ongoing education and training in culturally and linguistically appropriate service delivery.

STANDARD 4

Health care organizations must offer and provide language assistance services, including bilingual staff and interpreter services, at no cost to each patient/consumer with limited English proficiency at all points of contact, in a timely manner during all hours of operation.

STANDARD 5

Health care organizations must provide to patients/consumers in their preferred language both verbal offers and written notices informing them of their right to receive language assistance services.

STANDARD 6

Health care organizations must assure the competence of language assistance provided to limited English proficient patients/consumers by interpreters and bilingual staff. Family and friends should not be used to provide interpretation services (except on request by the patient/consumer).

STANDARD 7

Health care organizations must make available easily understood patient-related materials and post signage in the languages of the commonly encountered groups and/or groups represented in the service area.

STANDARD 8

Health care organizations should develop, implement, and promote a written strategic plan that outlines clear goals, policies, operational plans, and management accountability/oversight mechanisms to provide culturally and linguistically appropriate services.

STANDARD 9

Health care organizations should conduct initial and ongoing organizational self-assessments of CLAS-related activities and are encouraged to integrate cultural and linguistic competence-related measures into their internal audits, performance improvement programs, patient satisfaction assessments, and outcomes-based evaluations.

STANDARD 10

Health care organizations should ensure that data on the individual patient's/consumer's race, ethnicity, and spoken and written language are collected in health records, integrated into the organization's management information systems, and periodically updated.

STANDARD 11

Health care organizations should maintain a current demographic, cultural, and epidemiological profile of the community as well as a needs assessment to accurately plan for and implement services that respond to the cultural and linguistic characteristics of the service area.

STANDARD 12

Health care organizations should develop participatory, collaborative partnerships with communities and utilize a variety of formal and informal mechanisms to facilitate community and patient/consumer involvement in designing and implementing CLAS-related activities.

STANDARD 13

Health care organizations should ensure that conflict and grievance resolution processes are culturally and linguistically sensitive and capable of identifying, preventing, and resolving cross-cultural conflicts or complaints by patients/consumers.

STANDARD 14

Health care organizations are encouraged to regularly make available to the public information about their progress and successful innovations in implementing the CLAS standards and to provide public notice in their communities about the availability of this information.

NOTES

Introduction: My Fellow Humans

1. I would like to thank Michael Byrd and Linda Clayton for making their remarkable library available to me in preparation for this lecture, as well as for giving me the benefit of their learning and wisdom.

2. Soame Jenyns, "On the Chain of Universal Being," *Disquisitions on Several Subjects,* in *Works,* vol. 8, p. 231, quoted in A. O. Lovejoy, *The Great Chain of Being* (New York: Harper, 1960), p. 197.

3. See Stephen Jay Gould, *Ever Since Darwin* (New York: Norton, 1979), pp. 215–217.

4. Michael Byrd and Linda Clayton, *An American Health Dilemma,* vol. 1 (New York: Routledge, 2000), p. 218.

5. Quoted in Stephen Jay Gould, *The Flamingo's Smile* (New York: Norton, 1985), p. 296.

6. Byrd and Clayton, *Dilemma,* vol. 1, p. 163.

7. Thomas Jefferson, *Notes on the State of Virginia,* ed. William Peden (Chapel Hill: University of North Carolina Press, 1955), p. 163.

8. Quoted in Irv A. Brendlinger, *To Be Silent Would Be Criminal* (Lanham, MD: Scarecrow Press, 2007), p. 83.

1. It Takes a Village

1. Quoted in W. Montague Cobb, "The Black American in Medicine," *Journal of the National Medical Association* 73, supplement (December 1981), p. 1219.

2. Scrub Nurse

1. In 2008 I received an e-mail from Craig Sowell, the Delta Upsilon fraternity historian. He wrote that in 2001 he had interviewed Charles Prutzman, who had been the DU national president in

1956, the man who had canceled the convention. Prutzman, Sowell wrote, was 103 years old when he interviewed him, but still sharp. "In a life fully lived," Sowell had asked him, "do you have any major regrets?" Here is Prutzman's response: "The one thing that comes to mind that I would take back if I could . . . would be that I would *not* have canceled the 1956 convention. I did it out of pressure from the board members. But let's face it, it was a volatile time. Of course, if I knew then what I know now, I would never have made the decision the way I did. We did a horrible injustice, to an individual and to ourselves. But fortunately, the fence was mended a few years later."

3. Becoming a Doctor

1. Quoted in Emile Holman, "Sir William Osler, William Stewart Halsted, Harvey Cushing: Some Personal Reminiscences," *Surgery* 57 (1965), p. 595.

4. Becoming a Surgeon

1. Wayne Southwick, personal interview, September 15, 2008.
2. A. A. White et al., "Relief of Pain by Anterior Cervical Spine Fusion for Spondylosis: A Report of Sixty-Five Patients," *Journal of Bone and Joint Surgery* 55A (1973), pp. 525–534.

5. Combat Surgeon

1. When I came back from Vietnam in 1967, the epidemic of gunshot wounds in U.S. cities had become so severe that military surgeons were being sent into some big-city emergency rooms to teach debridement.
2. John Feagin, personal interview, October 20, 2008.
3. While working at the leprosarium I noticed what turned out to be an unknown disease. A number of patients had hands that were badly scarred. Much of the bone had simply been absorbed, while what was left showed severe disruption of the joints. Once I found that this syndrome had not been previously noted, I wrote it up and published it. A. A. White, "Disappearing Bone Disease with Ar-

thropathy and Severe Scarring of the Skin: A Report of Four Cases Seen in South Vietnam." *Journal of Bone and Joint Surgery* 53B (1971), pp. 303–309.

6. Getting toward Equal

1. Cobb, "Black American in Medicine," p. 1190.
2. R. W. Lovett, "The Mechanics of the Normal Spine and Its Relation to Scoliosis," *Medical and Surgical Journal* 153 (1905), p. 249, quoted in my thesis, *Analysis of the Mechanics of the Thoracic Spine in Man,* Acta Orthopaedica Scandinavica (Supplement 127) 1969, p. 8.

7. A Man Ain't Nothin' But a Man

1. See Allan Johnson, *Privilege, Power, and Difference* (New York: McGraw-Hill, 2006), and Tim Wise, *White Like Me* (Berkeley, CA: Softskull Press, 2008).

8. Orthopedic Chief

1. In earlier times, tattoo artists often mixed their inks with saliva, which created a pathway for infection. This is no longer the case.

9. Diagnosis and Treatment

1. Debra L. Roter and Judith A. Hall, *Doctors Talking with Patients / Patients Talking with Doctors* (Westport, CT: Praeger, 2006), p. 4.
2. Dan Goodenough, personal interview, January 29, 2009. Unless otherwise noted, all quotations from Goodenough are from this interview.
3. Pat Croskerry, "Achieving Quality in Clinical Decision Making: Cognitive Strategies for the Detection of Bias," *Academic Emergency Medicine* 9 (2002), p. 1198
4. Ibid.
5. Jerome Groopman, *How Doctors Think* (Boston: Houghton Mifflin, 2007), p. 40.
6. Ibid., p. 39.
7. Antonio Damasio, *Descartes' Error* (London: Penguin Books, 2005). In addition to Damasio, see, for example, Ronald de Sousa, *The*

Rationality of Emotion (Cambridge, MA: MIT Press, 1991), and Keith Oatley and P. N. Johnson-Laird, "Towards a Cognitive Theory of Emotion," *Cognition and Emotion* 1 (1987), pp. 29–50. Also, *How We Decide,* by the neuroscience writer Jonah Lehrer (Boston: Houghton Mifflin Harcourt, 2009).

8. Damasio, *Descartes' Error,* p. 185.

9. Ibid., pp. 159, 160.

10. See, for example, Diana Burgess et al., "Reducing Racial Bias among Health Care Providers: Lessons from Social-Cognitive Psychology," *Journal of General Internal Medicine* 22, no. 6 (June 2007), pp. 882–887.

11. David J. Schneider, *The Psychology of Stereotyping* (New York: Guilford Press, 2004), p. 564.

12. Ibid., p. 127.

13. *Focus,* January 9, 2004.

14. *Focus,* February 6, 2004.

15. Brian Smedley, Adrienne Stith, and Alan Nelson, eds., *Unequal Treatment: Confronting Racial and Ethnic Disparities in Health Care* (Washington, DC: Institute of Medicine, The National Academies Press, 2003).

10. Health-Care Disparities: Race

1. *Unequal Treatment,* pp. 38–79, 82. For infant mortality, see, e.g., Willie J. Parker, "Black-White Infant Mortality Disparity in the U.S.: A Social Litmus Test," *Public Health Reports* 118 (July–August 2003), pp. 336–337. For Harlem/Bangladesh comparison see C. McCord and H. P. Freeman, "Excess Mortality on Harlem," *New England Journal of Medicine* 332, no. 3 (January 18, 1990), pp. 173–177.

2. Alexander R. Green et al., "Implicit Bias among Physicians and Its Prediction of Thrombolysis Decisions for Black and White Patients," *Journal of Internal Medicine* 22, no. 9 (2007), pp. 1231–1238.

3. Lawrence D. Egbert and Irene L. Rothman, "Relation between the Race and Economic Status of Patients and Who Performs Their Surgery," *New England Journal of Medicine* 297, no. 2 (1971), pp. 90–91.

4. Knox H. Todd et al., "Ethnicity and Analgesic Practice," *Annals of Emergency Medicine* 35, no. 1 (January 2000), pp. 11–16.

5. In order to avoid using the cumbersome "he or she," we have alternated between the two throughout the book.

6. Knox H. Todd et al., "Ethnicity as a Risk Factor for Inadequate Emergency Department Analgesia," *Journal of the American Medical Association* 269, no. 12 (1993), pp. 1537–1539.

7. Vence L. Bonham, "Race, Ethnicity, and Pain Treatments: Striving to Understand the Causes and Solutions to the Disparities in Pain Treatments," *Journal of Law, Medicine, and Ethics* 29 (2001), pp. 52–68. Also see R. Sean Morrison et al., " 'We Don't Carry That'—Failure of Pharmacies in Predominantly Nonwhite Neighborhoods to Stock Opioid Analgesics," *New England Journal of Medicine* 342, no. 14 (April 6, 2000), pp. 1023–1026.

8. H. Jack Geiger, "Racial and Ethnic Disparities in Diagnosis and Treatment: A Review of the Evidence and a Consideration of Causes," in Smedley et al., *Unequal Treatment,* p. 425.

9. Alvin Poussaint, personal interview, February 18, 2009. Unless otherwise noted, all quotations from Poussaint are from this interview.

10. Schneider, *Psychology of Stereotyping,* pp. 96, 97.

11. Ibid., pp. 96, 97.

12. Ibid., p. 105. Also see Michelle Van Ryn and Jane Burke, "The Effect of Patient Race and Sex on Physician's Perception of Patients," *Social Science and Medicine* 50 (2000), pp. 813–828.

13. Mary-Jo Delvecchio Good et al., "The Culture of Medicine and Racial, Ethnic, and Class Disparities in Healthcare," in Smedley et al., *Unequal Treatment,* p. 603.

14. *Focus,* March 21, 2003.

15. Good et al., "Culture of Medicine," p. 595.

16. Joseph Betancourt, "Not Me! Doctors, Decisions, and Disparities in Health Care," *Cardiovascular Reviews and Reports,* May–June 2004, p. 106.

17. Good et al., "Culture of Medicine," p. 599.

18. Van Ryn and Burke, "Effect of Patient Race."

19. Roter and Hall, *Doctors Talking with Patients,* pp. 78–79.

20. Bruce Siegal, quoted in the *Wall Street Journal,* March 3, 2009, p. D1.

21. Harriet Washington, *Medical Apartheid* (New York: Doubleday, 2006).

22. "African Literature as Restoration and Celebration," quoted in the *New Yorker,* May 26, 2009, p. 74.

23. Robert Satcher did get his chemical engineering PhD from MIT and his MD from Harvard. He went on to become a board-certified orthopedic surgeon and musculoskeletal oncologist. After that he

was selected as a NASA astronaut. In November 2009 he was a member of the Atlantis crew on its mission to the International Space Station.

24. Erving Goffman, *Stigma* (Englewood Cliffs, NJ: Prentice-Hall, 1963), p. 14.

25. Damasio, *Descartes' Error,* pp. 256–257.

11. Health-Care Disparities: Women, Hispanics, Elderly, Gay

1. Kevin A. Schulman et al., "The Effect of Race and Sex on Physician's Recommendations for Cardiac Catheterization," *New England Journal of Medicine* 340, no. 8 (February 25, 1999), pp. 618–626.

2. It's interesting to note that Claudia practices with four African American male orthopedic surgeons, all of whom had been her students, in a partnership that serves a mainly white Florida community.

3. Claudia Thomas, personal interview, January 18, 2009. Unless otherwise noted, all quotations from Thomas are from this interview.

4. R. Di Cecco et al., "Is There a Clinically Significant Gender Bias in Post-Myocardial Infarction Pharmacological Management in the Older Population of a Primary Care Practice?" *BioMed Central Family Practice* 3 (2002), p. 8. Also, Hani Jneid et al., "Sex Difference in Medical Care and Early Death after Acute Myocardial Infarction," *Circulation* 118 (2008), pp. 2803–2810.

5. Thomas Concannon et al., "Elapsed Time in Emergency Medical Services for Patients with Cardiac Complaints," *Circulation* (online), January 13, 2009.

6. There is speculation that EMT time regarding women is due to confusion about symptoms.

7. Jneid, "Sex Difference."

8. Gabrielle Chiaramonte, "Physicians' Gender Bias in the Diagnosis, Treatment, and Interpretation of Coronary Heart Disease Symptoms," paper presented at the 20th Annual Conference of the Transcatheter Cardiovascular Research Foundation.

9. Dorry Segev et al., "Age and Comorbidities Are Effect Modifiers of Gender Disparities in Renal Transplantation," *Journal of the American Society of Nephrology* (online), January 7, 2009.

10. Cornelia M. Borkhoff et al., "The Effect of Patients' Sex on Physicians' Recommendations for Total Knee Arthroplasty," *Canadian Medical Association Journal* (online), March 11, 2008 (6), p. 178.

11. Mary O'Connor, personal interview, February 16, 2009. Unless otherwise noted, all quotations from O'Connor are from this interview.

12. Richard Currey, "Ageism in Healthcare: Time for a Change," *Aging Well* 1, no. 1 (Winter 2008), p. 16.

13. John Rowe, personal interview, April 9, 2009. Unless otherwise noted, all quotes from Rowe are from this interview.

14. Becca Levy et al., "Longevity Increases by Positive Self-Perceptions of Aging," *Journal of Personality and Social Psychology* 83, no. 2 (2002), pp. 261–270.

15. Ibid., p. 268.

16. Daniel Callahan, "New Old Age Blog," *New York Times,* November 13, 2008.

17. Smedley et al., *Unequal Treatment,* Literature Review, pp. 285–383. Also S. Saha, editorial, *Journal of General Internal Medicine* 22, Supplement 2 (2007), pp. 371–372.

18. Eric Cheng et al., "Primary Language and Receipt of Recommended Health Care among Hispanics in the United States," *Journal of General Internal Medicine* 22, Supplement 2 (November 2007), pp. 283–288.

19. Joseph Betancourt, personal interview, March 5, 2009.

20. Ibid.

21. Leonor Fernandez, personal interview, February 23, 2009. Unless otherwise noted, all quotations from Fernandez are from this interview.

22. Betancourt, "Not Me!," p. 106.

23. Joseph Kramer, personal interview, March 13, 2009.

24. Ibid.

25. Harvey Makadon, personal interview, February 22, 2009. Unless otherwise noted, all quotations from Makadon are from this interview.

26. Harvey Makadon, "Improving Health Care for Lesbian and Gay Communities," *New England Journal of Medicine* 354, no. 9 (March 2, 2006), p. 895.

27. Harvey Makadon et al., "Optimizing Primary Care for Men Who Have Sex with Men," *Journal of the American Medical Association* 296, no. 19 (November 15, 2006), p. 2363.

28.   Gregorio Millet et al., "Focusing Down-Low: Black Men, HIV Risk, and Heterosexual Transmission," *Journal of the National Medical Association* 97, no. 7, Supplement (July 2005), pp. 52s–59s.

12. Culturally Competent Care

1.   Somnath Saha et al., "Patient Centeredness, Cultural Competence, and Health Care Quality," *Journal of the National Medical Association* 100, no. 11 (November 2008), pp. 1275–1285.

2.   Leonor Fernandez, personal interview, February 23, 2009. Unless otherwise noted, all quotations from Fernandez are from this interview.

3.   Thomas A. Laveist, "Is Doctor-Patient Race Concordance Associated with Greater Satisfaction with Care?" *Journal of Health and Social Behavior* 43, no. 3 (September 2002), pp. 296–306.

4.   Moira Stewart, "Effective Physician-Patient Communication and Health Outcomes: A Review," *Journal of the Canadian Medical Association* 152, no. 9 (May 1, 1955), pp. 1423–1431; Moira Stewart et al., "The Impact of Patient-Centered Care on Outcomes," *Journal of Family Practice* 49, no. 9 (September 2000), pp. 796–804; Lisa Cooper and Debra Roter, "Patient-Provider Communication: The Effect of Race and Ethnicity on Process and Outcomes of Healthcare," in Smedley et al., *Unequal Treatment*, pp. 552–579.

5.   Richard Street et al., "Understanding Concordance in Patient-Physician Relationships: Personal and Ethnic Dimensions of Shared Identity," *Annals of Family Medicine* 6 (2008), pp. 198–205. Also see Gloria Bonner et al., "Determinants of Trust and Mistrust in Physicians Identified by African American Caregivers," *African American Research Perspectives* 11 (2005), pp. 89–102.

6.   Street et al., "Understanding Concordance."

7.   Lisa Cooper et al., "Delving below the Surface: Understanding How Race and Ethnicity Influence Relationships in Health Care," *Journal of General Internal Medicine* 21, Supplement 1 (January 21, 2006), pp. S21–S27.

8.   Roter and Hall, *Doctors Talking with Patients*, p. 58.

9.   At the same time, an expectation of distance, unease, or suspicion will tend to elicit distance, unease, and suspicion. I will never forget

the vignette a psychiatry professor of mine at Stanford told us. Dr. Seymour Kolko recounted that when he was an intern he was working in the locked ward at a psychiatric institution. There was a violent patient in this ward who continually rejected his food, knocking the food trays around and physically attacking the attendants delivering them. Dr. Kolko spent a good deal of time trying to establish rapport with this patient, and eventually he got to the point where he thought he himself would be able to deliver a food tray safely. He approached the door of the patient's room, spoke softly to him, and reminded him of their previous friendly discussions. After many minutes of preparation, Dr. Kolko felt ready. He picked up the tray, took his glasses off and put them in his pocket, approached the patient slowly and in as nonthreatening a manner as he could, and . . . bam! The patient unleashed a powerful uppercut, sending dishes and food flying. Then he went after Dr. Kolko himself. Afterward Kolko understood his mistake. In taking off his glasses he had signaled that he expected violence, and violence was what he got.

10. Roxana Llerena-Quinn, personal interview, May 1, 2009.

11. Ibid.

12. Kenneth Harvey and Tracy Lazloffy, "The Cultural Genogram: Key to Training Culturally Competent Family Therapists," *Journal of Marital and Family Therapy* 21, no. 3 (1995), pp. 227–237.

13. E. J. Langer et al., "Decreasing Prejudice by Increasing Discrimination," *Journal of Personal Social Psychology* 49, no. 1 (July 1985), pp. 113–120.

14. Maja Djikic et al., "Reducing Stereotyping through Mindfulness: Effects on Automatic Stereotype-Activated Behavior," *Journal of Adult Development* 15 (2008), pp. 106–111.

15. Diana Burgess et al., "Reducing Racial Bias among Health Care Providers: Lessons from Social-Cognitive Psychology," *Journal of General Internal Medicine* 22, no. 6 (June 2007), pp. 882–887.

16. Schneider, *Psychology of Stereotyping*, pp. 376–433. Also see Irene Blaire, "The Malleability of Automatic Stereotypes and Prejudice," *Personality and Social Psychology Review* 6, no. 3 (2002), pp. 247–261.

17. Dean K. Whitla et al., "Educational Benefits of Diversity in Medical School: A Survey of Students," *Academic Medicine* 78, no. 5 (May 2003), pp. 460–466.

18. United States Census Bureau, Population Estimates, Available at http://www.census.gov/popest/estimates.php.

19. The [Louis] Sullivan Commission, *Missing Persons: Minorities in the Health Professions,* Executive Summary, p. 2.

20. Ibid., p. 1.

21. Steven Woolf et al., "The Health Impact of Resolving Racial Disparities: An Analysis of U.S. Mortality Data," *American Journal of Public Health* 94, no. 12 (December 2004), pp. 278–281. Also see David Satcher et al., "What If We Were Equal? A Comparison of the Black-White Mortality Gap in 1960 and 2000," *Health Affairs* 24, no. 2 (2005), pp. 459–464.

22. African Americans; Appalachian poor; Asian Americans; the elderly; gay, lesbian, bisexual, transgendered; immigrants; Hispanics; Native Americans; the obese; various religious groups; women; those other than normally abled; and prisoners. Prisoners are not strictly part of this group in that it would be hard to argue that they should have access to the same high level of care as minority groups should, but do not, enjoy. I am including them here because they are often denied even a basic level of decent, humane medical treatment. I've used the phrase "those other than normally abled" because, though cumbersome, it avoids both the illogic of the more common "alternately abled" and the pejorative of "disabled."

23. Thanks to Michael Byrd for this thought.

24. Tait Shanafelt et al., "Career Fit and Burnout among Academic Faculty," *Archives of Internal Medicine* 169, no. 10 (May 25, 2009), pp. 990–995.

Epilogue

1. See Phillip Goff et al., "Not Yet Human: Implicit Knowledge, Historical Dehumanization, and Contemporary Consequences," *Journal of Personality and Social Psychology* 94, no. 2 (2008), pp. 292–306.

2. See, for example, E. D. Hirsch, *Cultural Literacy* (Boston: Houghton Mifflin, 1987).

3. Multicultural awareness and education is, for instance, exemplified in the courses and programs of Professor James A. Banks at the University of Washington.

4. See Camara Jones, "Levels of Racism: A Theoretic Framework and a Gardener's Tale," *American Journal of Public Health* 90, no. 8 (2000), pp. 1212–1215.

5. Leon Eisenberg, "From Affirmative Action to Transformative Research," *The Word Connection*, February 2008.

6. Derek Bok and William Bowen, *The Shape of the River* (Princeton: Princeton University Press, 2000).

7. R. C. Davidson and E. L. Lewis, "Affirmative Action and Other Special Consideration Admissions at the University of California, Davis School of Medicine," *Journal of the American Medical Association* 278, no. 14 (October 8, 1997) pp. 1153–1158.

8. Adam Liptak, "The Waves Minority Judges Always Make," *New York Times*, May 31, 2009.

9. Thanks to Leon Eisenberg for bringing this quote to my attention.

10. Johnson, *Privilege, Power, and Difference*, p. 153.

ACKNOWLEDGMENTS

First, I can never say enough about my tremendous gratitude for the collaboration with David Chanoff on this project. In the course of research and writing we became true colleagues and warm friends, which was an additional and invaluable benefit beyond the satisfaction of bringing these experiences and ideas into book form.

I also want to acknowledge and thank Blue Cross Blue Shield of Massachusetts, the Macy Foundation, the J. Robert Gladden Orthopedic Society, and the Arthur and Barbara Higgins Charitable Foundation for generous support in the preparation of this book.

In addition, I wish to express my deep appreciation to a number of my fellow humans who have helped in a variety of ways to make this work possible. Since I am a person who thrives on the creative input and feedback of friends, colleagues, and family, the list is a long one. Some of the following people helped through reading and commenting on chapters, others through advice on specific topics, and others through more general discussions of the large social, medical, and scientific issues we have addressed. My thanks for these gifts go to Verona Brewton, Wayne Budd, Dr. Michael Byrd, Liisa Chanoff, Dr. Marni Chanoff, Dr. Linda Clayton, Dr. Malcolm Cox, Rabbi Aaron Fine, Dr. Gary and Linda Friedlender, Dr. Harris Gibson, Dr. James Hill, Matthew Hills, Dr. Sandra Holly, Dr. James Hoyte, Dr. Peter Jokl, Cleve Killingsworth, Dr. Gerard Lawrence, Dean Daniel Lowenstein, Buzz and Mava Luttrell, Dr. Henrik Malchau, Dean Joseph Martin, Alanna Maurais, Lucrecia McClure, John and Beverly McDaniels, Barry Merkin, Rose Ann Miller, Dr. and Mrs. Randall Morgan, Jr., Jodi Nagel, Charles Ogletree, Dr. Nancy Oriol, Dr. Manohar Panjabi, Dr. Chet Pierce, Dr. Ray Pierce, Dr. Giuseppe Raviola, Dr. Joan Reede, Emily Rickards, Terttu Savoie, Alane Shanks,

Ray Shepard, Dr. Helen Shields, Dr. Bill Taylor, Dr. Samuel Thier, Tyson Tildon, Dr. Bill Tipton, Rabbi Avram Turin, Robin Waxenberg, Peter H. Weis, Dr. Carlton West, Alissa White, Anita White, Annica White, Arnett White, Atina White, and Dr. Mike Yaszemski.

Among those who have contributed to this project I would like especially to thank my medical colleagues who graciously agreed to formal interviews, some of which appeared in the book, some which didn't, but all of which helped us convey a feel for the way inequalities affect the hands-on practice of medicine. These colleagues are Drs. Joseph Betancourt, John Feagin, Leonor Fernandez, Daniel Goodenough, Douglas Jackson, Joseph Kramer, Roxana Llerena-Quinn, Harvey Makadon, Mary O'Connor, Alvin Poussaint, Laurie Raymond, Wayne Southwick and Mrs. Ann Southwick, and Claudia Thomas.

I am not sure if it is common for authors to mention the people who served as inspirations for them as they progressed through their writing and especially through the real work of living and wrestling with the experiences and ideas that lead up to writing. But for me, those people have been very much in my mind during the course of bringing this book to fruition. These individuals have contributed in a variety of major ways in my life as mentors, mentees, or role models. Some I have known very well, some slightly, others only indirectly, but to all of them I feel the need to acknowledge my debt: Muhammad Ali, Dr. Mark Bernhardt, Dr. Henry Bohlman, Jim Brown, Coach Vincent A. Campbell, Dr. Montague Cobb, Dr. Alvin Crawford, Dr. Paul Curtis, the Dalai Lama, Anthony Davids, Michael Dukakis, Dr. Daryll Dykes, Dr. Charles Epps, Dr. Mark Gebhardt, Dorothy Height, Dr. Carl Hirsch, Daniel Hogan, Dr. Marshall Holley, Langston Hughes, Paul Johnson, Addie Jones, C. S. (Doc) Jones, K. C. and Ellen Jones, Dr. Don King, Dr. Martin Luther King, Jr., Malcolm X, Nelson Mandela, Dr. Henry Mankin, Dr. Alf Nachemson, Rev. Willie Naulls, Barack Obama, Dr. Don Prolo, Ted Parrish, Dr. Preston Phillips, Dr. Anthony Rankin, Coach Joe Restic, Dr. Victor Richards, Bill Russell, Dr. Bertil Stener, Dr. Louis Sullivan,

Charles Tarpley, Dean Daniel Tosteson, and my mother and father, Vivian and Augustus White, Jr.

There are others who have been enormously helpful who are not listed here. I trust they will know I am grateful, accept the expression of my appreciation, and forgive the omission. Zach Alexander was my administrative assistant through most of the writing, and Yolanda Bauer provided similar assistance toward the end of the project. I am grateful to both of them for their efficiency, thoroughness, and unfailing good humor in what was sometimes a challenging process.

Finally, my thanks go to Ann Downer-Hazell, who saw enough value in this project to acquire it for Harvard University Press, and to Elizabeth Knoll, who provided guidance and editorial wisdom throughout our endeavors.

INDEX